THE PSYCHOLOGY OF RUNNING

Why do people run? How can I improve my running performance? Will running help me feel better?

The Psychology of Running provides a unique insight into why running is such a popular form of exercise and competition. From evolutionary perspectives on why humans have needed to run and how our bodies have adapted for this function, to discussing evidence-based interventions that can improve running performance, the book delves into the psychological motivations and benefits of running. The book also considers ways in which running can be used for social change and life skill development, highlighting how such a simple activity can have benefits for our physical and mental health.

Providing proven psychological strategies and techniques to help improve running performance and boost our individual self-belief, *The Psychology of Running* shows us how we can enjoy running, no matter our age or ability.

Noel Brick, PhD, is a lecturer in sport and exercise psychology at Ulster University in Ireland. He is a chartered psychologist with the British Psychological Society and a registered sport and exercise psychologist with the Health and Care Professions Council (HCPC). He has applied his experience as a sport and exercise psychologist in a range of performance settings including running, cycling, powerlifting, and Gaelic games. Noel's research interests include the psychology of endurance performance, with an emphasis on the psychology of long-distance running. His research also focuses on mental health in sport. Noel has completed over 30 marathons and ultramarathons, including the Marathon des Sables in 2012 and the Boston Marathon in 2022. Noel is also co-author of *The Genius of Athletes*.

Stuart Holliday is a chartered psychologist with the British Psychological Society and a registered sport and exercise psychologist with the Health and Care Professions Council (HCPC) based in London. He has worked for over ten years in the field with Olympic, Paralympic, and Premiership squads and teams. His main interest is in endurance sports, and running in particular. He works in private practice with athletes at all competitive levels and is a keen club runner, competing across all distances up to the marathon. Stuart was a contributing author to *Touring and Mental Health: The Music Industry Manual*.

THE PSYCHOLOGY OF EVERYTHING

People are fascinated by psychology, and what makes humans tick. Why do we think and behave the way we do? We've all met armchair psychologists claiming to have the answers, and people that ask if psychologists can tell what they're thinking. *The Psychology of Everything* is a series of books which debunk the popular myths and pseudo-science surrounding some of life's biggest questions.

The series explores the hidden psychological factors that drive us, from our subconscious desires and aversions, to our natural social instincts. Absorbing, informative, and always intriguing, each book is written by an expert in the field, examining how research-based knowledge compares with popular wisdom, and showing how psychology can truly enrich our understanding of modern life.

Applying a psychological lens to an array of topics and contemporary concerns—from sex, to fashion, to conspiracy theories—*The Psychology of Everything* will make you look at everything in a new way.

Titles in the series:

The Psychology of Art
by George Mather

The Psychology of Wellness
by Gary W. Wood

The Psychology of Comedy
by G Neil Martin

The Psychology of Democracy
by Darren G. Lilleker and Billur Aslan Ozgul

The Psychology of Counselling
by Marie Percival

The Psychology of Travel
by Andrew Stevenson

The Psychology of Attachment
by Robbie Duschinsky, Pehr Granqvist and Tommie Forslund

The Psychology of Running
by Noel Brick and Stuart Holliday

For more information about this series, please visit: www.routledge textbooks.com/textbooks/thepsychologyofeverything/

THE PSYCHOLOGY OF RUNNING

NOEL BRICK AND STUART HOLLIDAY

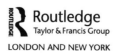

Routledge
Taylor & Francis Group

LONDON AND NEW YORK

Designed cover image: © Getty Images

First published 2024
by Routledge
4 Park Square, Milton Park, Abingdon, Oxon OX14 4RN

and by Routledge
605 Third Avenue, New York, NY 10158

Routledge is an imprint of the Taylor & Francis Group, an informa business

British Library Cataloguing-in-Publication Data
A catalogue record for this book is available from the British Library

ISBN: 978-1-032-06862-6 (hbk)
ISBN: 978-1-032-06861-9 (pbk)
ISBN: 978-1-003-20420-6 (ebk)

DOI: 10.4324/9781003204206

Typeset in Joanna
by Apex CoVantage, LLC

CONTENTS

ACKNOWLEDGEMENTS

We would first like to thank the team at Routledge for giving us the opportunity to write this book and for their support and encouragement along the way. Writing this book with you was an enjoyable experience. Thank you for your patience!

We would like to thank some people that we interviewed for this book and the runners who were willing to share their experiences of working with us. Many of their stories helped to shape the Run with it sections at the end of specific chapters. We extend this thanks to Allie Riley, Deborah Pleva, Beth Gordon, and Dillon McClintock for providing fantastic insights into the Girls on the Run programme, and to Kirsty Woodbridge for her insights into parkrun. And to "Angela," "Chris," and "Russell" for their contributions to case studies within this book. We are also grateful to Holly Brick and Roisin Bolger, who reviewed earlier versions of this book and provided invaluable feedback to make it better.

We would like to thank those who have shaped our educational journey, provided mentorship, and helped to develop us as academics and practitioners capable of writing a book like The Psychology of Running. We hope we have done you some justice. Noel would like to thank Dr P.J. Smith, Dr Mark Campbell, Dr Tadhg MacIntyre, and Prof Stewart Cotterill. Stuart would like to thank Prof Andy Lane, Dan

Robinson, Dr Caroline Marlow, and running coach and friend Steve Hobbs for their insight and wisdom on all matters psychology and running.

Finally, we would like to thank our families for their patience and support throughout the journey of writing this book. The time spent sitting at a desk, tapping on a keyboard, would not have been possible without you. Noel would like to thank Holly for her support, for listening to him bounce many ideas around, for her good advice to improve these ideas, and for the umpteen cups of tea and coffee. He would also like to thank his mum and dad, P.J., Thomas, Mary, and each of his extended family members for their unending kindness, encouragement, and support. Stuart would like to thank his parents for encouraging him to try out new things, and especially Lucy and Herbie, who have always supported him in his work, study, and play and for being there every step of the way.

INTRODUCTION

We love to run! We are two of millions of people around the world for whom running is a central part of their lives. Running has brought us on a life journey that, for both Noel and Stuart, has not only provided a recreational and competitive outlet, but has also become a fundamental part of our working lives. We owe a lot to running and we hope that we give something back by sharing the many insights we have learned through our research, applied practice, and running activity over the past 20+ years.

This book aims to provide an overview of The Psychology of Running from a number of different perspectives. Each chapter will be structured around a central question like: Why do we run? Why do we slow down or stop? What can we think about to run faster, and what can we focus on to make running feel easier and more pleasant? Aside from performance-related topics, we will also provide evidence-based answers to questions such as: Can running help me feel better? And, what can running teach adults and children about life?

Within The Psychology of Running, Chapter 1 will provide some answers to a basic, fundamental question: Why do we run? The answers will include a brief overview of running behaviour from an evolutionary perspective and explore how early humans used running to meet their basic survival needs. We will consider how running has shaped

DOI: 10.4324/9781003204206-1

the physical structure of our body. More importantly, this chapter will also argue that the need to simultaneously run, navigate our environment, make decisions, and switch our attention between various sources of information provided the ideal stimulus for the human brain to adapt and evolve. We will also highlight the importance of different motives that explain why we continue to run today even though, in reality, we don't necessarily have to.

Chapter 2 will provide an overview of research on the psychological factors that determine running performance. These include our motivation to run and how easy or hard running feels. Evidence for other psychological factors important to running performance and longer-term running behaviour will be presented, including exercise-induced pain, how good or bad we feel during running, and the strength of our beliefs about what we are capable of as runners. This chapter will also spotlight some research that has highlighted the negative impact of psychological factors, like mental fatigue, on running performance.

Chapter 3 will build on Chapter 2 and present an overview of evidence-based psychological interventions that help improve running performance. Within this, we will discuss which psychological techniques can help us to run faster or keep going for longer distances. These evidence-based techniques include goal setting, what we say to ourselves (our self-talk), relaxation techniques, and mental imagery. This chapter will conclude by providing a real-world case study from a runner we worked with to highlight how these psychological techniques can be used to improve your own running performance.

Chapter 4 will provide an overview of research on the effects of our focus of attention on running outcomes. This chapter will not only present research on the impact of attentional focus on running performance, but also evidence of the effects of different strategies on how easy or hard a run feels, and on how good or bad we feel when running. These are important because running isn't only about running faster, it is also about feeling better and enjoying what we do, both important outcomes to help us sustain longer-term running behaviour. In this chapter we will also provide insight into psychological techniques that help increase running enjoyment.

In Chapter 5, we will provide an overview of the mental health and brain health benefits that running can bring and provide practical suggestions on parameters to optimise these benefits, including the frequency, intensity, and duration of running required to gain mental health benefits. Importantly, this discussion aims to dispel the myth that we need to train like a marathon runner to improve our mental health. Instead, this chapter will provide evidence that as little as 10 minutes of jogging can enhance our post-run mood. Despite being a relatively simple activity, running also challenges our brain in many ways and the existing evidence suggests that the mental demands imposed by running result in many positive adaptations to our brain, including improvements in memory, attention, and enhanced connections in regions of our brain involved in these mental processes. These findings suggest that running can improve brain health across our lifespan and has the potential to protect our brain from age-related decline and dementia. We will also learn in Chapter 5 that, despite the many benefits, there is also a darker side to running. We will conclude Chapter 5 with some insights into running addiction and provide a tool to help you screen your own risk for addiction to running.

Finally, Chapter 6 will build on Chapter 5 and introduce evidence on how running has been used as a vehicle for social change and life skill development. This chapter will focus on running-based initiatives aimed at school children and adults in community settings. With school children, we will focus on the psychological outcomes associated with two programmes, The Daily Mile and Girls on the Run. The Daily Mile is a school-based initiative that aims to provide children with a 15-minute bout of running, walking, or wheeling during each school day. Evidence suggests that The Daily Mile can have benefits for children's physical and mental health. Adopting running for a different reason, Girls on the Run uses a 10-week programme as a vehicle to build confidence, develop relationships, and teach life skills to 8-to-14-year-old girls in the U.S.A. and Canada. Recent evaluations of the programme highlight positive outcomes, such as an improved ability to regulate emotions and increased confidence among girls who take part in the programme.

Chapter 6 will also introduce running-based initiatives that are focused on teenagers and adults. We will present several initiatives that use running to help homeless people or those at risk of homelessness. These include The Running Charity, Back on My Feet, and A Mile in Her Shoes. Each of these programmes aims to foster connection and provide social support for programme participants. In addition, the available evidence indicates that these programmes help participants feel more self-sufficient and provides a boost to their self-esteem and self-confidence. Finally, will also present an overview of research on parkrun, a free, weekly, community-based 5km event that takes place in locations throughout the world. parkrun research has highlighted many mental and social health benefits for those who take part. These include better mental health, a sense of achievement when completing a parkrun event, greater social connection and interaction, and higher satisfaction with one's life overall. Importantly, because it is free to participate in, parkrun also helps to reduce the social inequalities that often prove a barrier to physical activity behaviour.

Within Chapters 2 to 6, we also include a "Run with it" section at the end of each chapter. These sections provide you with a clearer insight into how you can adopt many of the psychological techniques and strategies presented in the book to help build your self-belief as a runner (Chapter 2), to improve your running performance (Chapter 3), or to increase your running enjoyment (Chapter 4). In Chapter 5, we provide a tool to screen for your risk of exercise addiction. Finally, we provide a deeper insight into Girls on the Run in Chapter 6 to give a first-hand account of the short- and longer-term benefits associated with taking part in that programme.

We hope you enjoy reading this book—and learning from it—as much as we enjoyed writing it. Each of the strategies and outcomes that we present in this book are based on an evidence base of good-quality scientific research that we have attempted to distil in a clear and accessible way. Whatever your reasons are for reading it, we hope this book will help you in the long run.

1

WHY DO WE RUN?

INTRODUCTION

Running is not a uniquely human behaviour. However, what is relatively unique is our capability, and our motivation, to run for long distances. Few other species, apart from some breeds of dog, run such long distances. Running is one of the most popular forms of leisure time physical activity worldwide, and statistics from both Europe and the U.S.A. estimate that the number of people who run is more than 50 million in each region (Rizzo, 2021; Scheerder et al., 2015). In competitive race events, global participation was estimated to have peaked at 9.1 million race finishers in 2016 (Anderson, 2021).

Each of these figures point to the popularity of running as a form of physical activity. But why is this the case? Why do we run? Perhaps to begin to explain why running is so popular today, we first need to go back to the very beginning and answer a fundamental question about human evolution: Why do humans run?

WHY DO HUMANS RUN?

There are, of course, many running intensities, ranging from slow jogging to maximal sprinting. When scientists first explored humans' sprinting capabilities, their broad conclusion was that humans, by

DOI: 10.4324/9781003204206-2

comparison with other species, are pretty abysmal runners. The current 100-meter world record for men of 9.58 seconds, set by Usain Bolt at the 2009 World Athletics Championships, equates to an average running speed of 37.58km per hour. Bolt achieved a peak sprinting speed of 44.72km per hour during that race. By comparison, a cheetah, the fastest land animal on Earth, can reach a top speed of approximately 112km per hour. Greyhounds and thoroughbred horses can both race around a track at approximately 70km per hour. Even the average family cat, with little training or skin-tight clothing to minimise wind resistance, could outsprint the fastest human on Earth with its 48km per hour maximum running speed. It's humbling (and equally terrifying) to consider that—if it so desired—your cat could outsprint you.

For generations, our deficiencies as sprinters over short distances led many scientists to ignore our potential as runners. Instead, the evolution of the human body shape, with long limbs and an upright posture, combined with a relatively slow sprinting capacity, was taken as evidence that the primary form of locomotion that shaped human evolution was walking. Sprinting was the forte of predators that, like cheetahs and other cats, rely on speed and agility to hunt.

But sprinting isn't the only form of running. One niche that humans do specialise in is running at slower speeds over considerable distances. When comparisons are made using endurance running—defined as running for distances beyond five kilometres using aerobic metabolism—then humans fare much better. The average speed of a recreational jogger, which is anywhere between 8.2km and 15.0km per hour over the course of 42.2km marathon, means that we outperform many other animals, such as hunting dogs, hyenas, wildebeest, and horses over longer distances. Many features of the human body also help us run more efficiently for extended periods. This leads to a second set of questions: Were humans built to run long distances? Or did long-distance running shape the evolution of the human form that we have today? Much evidence suggests that the latter may be the case.

DID LONG-DISTANCE RUNNING SHAPE THE HUMAN BODY?

The idea that long-distance running helped shape human evolution has been around since the early 1980s (Carrier, 1984). But in 2004, biologist Dennis Bramble and paleoanthropologist Daniel Lieberman considered how endurance running impacted the shape and structure of many parts of the human body. Our long Achilles tendons and elastic foot arches, for example, act like springs and propel us forward during running, but not during walking. Relatively short toes reduce the amount of energy required to stabilise our foot during ground contact in running and, by doing so, mean that every stride we take is more efficient than species with longer toes, such as apes (Rolian et al., 2009). When we walk, however, shorter toes make little difference to the amount of energy expended. Our large and sturdy ankle, knee, and hip joints help to dissipate the forces generated each time our running feet strike the ground. Large gluteus maximus muscles help us run at all speeds, but contribute little to walking, suggesting that the enlargement of this muscle was more important to our evolution as runners than as walkers (Lieberman et al., 2006).

These running-specific adaptations continue in our upper body. Our tall waist, flexible spine, and wide shoulders allow us to counter-rotate our trunk relative to our hips during the flight phase of running, when both feet leave the ground. A flight phase only happens during running, whereas in walking, one foot is always in contact with the ground. (This flight phase is what differentiates race walking from running.) The configuration of muscles in our back, shoulders, and neck, coupled with a large semi-circular canal system in our inner ear, also allows us to stabilise our upper-body, head, and, crucially, our gaze when the movement of our lower limbs might otherwise throw us off balance (Spoor et al., 1994). Finally, to cool down when we run, our long, relatively hairless bodies, coupled with an abundance of sweat glands in our skin, means that we have a large surface area capable of dissipating heat relatively quickly. As a result, while many other running mammals, such as hunting dogs and hyenas, are constrained to run during cooler dusk, night-time, or dawn temperatures, humans alone are capable of long-distance running in hot daytime temperatures. This competitive advantage most likely allowed early humans to use persistence hunting, and specifically endurance running during hot, daytime temperatures to drive prey into hyperthermia and exhaustion (Lieberman et al., 2006).

To provide one answer to the question of why humans run long distances is that running may have allowed our early ancestors to fill a niche position as daytime carnivores. Being capable of running long distances relatively quickly during daytime hours meant that we could scavenge the carcasses of prey long before other running scavengers, like hyenas, arrived to pick the bones. In time, being able to run and thermoregulate effectively in daytime temperatures also meant that we could use persistence hunting as a strategy, forcing our prey to run at a high and, for them, inefficient speed until the animal eventually overheated and collapsed from exhaustion. Although running for long periods might seem like a strategy that requires a lot of energy, the rewards of a protein-dense and calorie-rich meal more than compensated for the costs. As such, better runners held a competitive advantage that shaped the evolution of the human body over the generations that followed.

HOW DID RUNNING IMPACT OUR BRAIN?

While these accounts may help to explain why humans run, and the impact of running on the evolution of our physical form, perhaps less obvious is the profound impact running had on the evolution of our brain. The human brain is about three times bigger than might be expected for our body size (Lieberman, 2011). Increased brain size became most pronounced about 2 million years ago in a species of archaic human called *Homo erectus* (meaning "upright man"), considered to be the first human ancestor to shift to a hunting, gathering, and scavenging lifestyle. The increase in brain size is often attributed to the increased complexity of the social world and physical environment of *Homo erectus*. Our ancestors were, and we still are, social animals, and living and hunting in groups required communication and collaboration with others. Similarly, exploring their surroundings, finding the safest places to live, or scouring the most bountiful hunting grounds stimulated other brain activities, or what psychologists call *cognitive functions*, such as focused attention, multi-tasking, planning, decision-making, and both short- and long-term memory. While the requirements of our social world impacted the evolution of our brain, evidence also suggests that the increased size of our ancestors' brain occurred at the same time as their physical activity levels increased (Bramble & Lieberman, 2004). In other words, bigger brains may have been the result of a much more physically active lifestyle that involved hunting, gathering, and, of course, running.

But how and why did running lead to a bigger brain in humans? Perhaps more importantly, how and why does physical exercise like running continue to impact our brain structure and function today? One idea, called the Adaptive Capacity Model (Raichlen & Alexander, 2017), helps to explain why physical activities like running can lead to improved brain structure and function. When we think about it, our prehistoric ancestors didn't just run about aimlessly. Instead, they ran with a hunter-gatherer focus, foraging for food as they navigated their environment. Not only were they physically active, early humans were also cognitively active when they roamed their environment.

Even at the most basic level, running, in and of itself, poses a challenge for our brain to coordinate and control the movements of our body. But running as a forager is more complex and creates additional mental demands. Much like modern-day orienteering, our forebears needed to navigate their environment, choosing the best path across open habitats and over uneven terrain. New, unexplored, and unfamiliar territories made these tasks harder. Our ancestors also needed to pay attention to their surroundings, shift their attention from one object to the next, and process relevant information about those objects, like whether there are berries on a nearby tree, or whether the mound in the distance is a clump of dry grass or a predator waiting to pounce. Successful foragers might also use their memory of past experiences to know where the richest sources of food might be found, to remember how to navigate to these locations, or to know whether a bunch of berries were edible or poisonous. Stalking prey might have proven even more physically and mentally demanding, running at a suitable pace while simultaneously tracking footprints on the ground, monitoring an animal's movements, continually shifting attention from prey to the environment, communicating with other hunters in their pack, and using memories of previous efforts to plan the best means to capture a prey. Over a lifetime, each of the demands of a hunter-gatherer existence challenged our brain, stimulated it to adapt, and, in turn, increased its capacity to perform the cognitive functions required for successful outcomes.

These ideas go some way to explain why movement is so important to the health of our brain. Humans adapted to a physical lifestyle that consisted of large amounts of mentally effortful, moderate-intensity activity. We did not adapt to the relatively inactive and sedentary lifestyle that many of us lead today. By maintaining a physically active lifestyle, we continue to challenge our brains in a similar way as our ancestors did and, by doing so, help to increase or maintain the structure and function of our brain as we grow older. Evidence to support this idea comes from the many studies that show that aerobic exercise, like running, leads to the growth of new neurons, or nerve cells within the brain, and results in better connectivity between existing neurons. In turn, these adaptations are linked with better performance on mental tasks that require attention, multi-tasking, decision-making, and memory, for example (Colcombe & Kramer, 2003). Adding mental challenges to our physical activity can provide an additional boost. One recent study, for example, found that orienteering experts reported greater spatial memory abilities (that is, memory of information about locations, like being able to navigate your way through streets in a town) than non-orienteering, physically active counterparts; meaning that the physical and mental demands of a sport like orienteering can provide an additional stimulus to maintain our mental abilities (Waddington & Heisz, 2023). These benefits of running are something we will explore in much more detail in Chapter 5, where we will provide an insight into the effects of running on both our mental health and on the health of our brain.

Mechanisms provided by models like the Adaptive Capacity Model also help us to understand why long periods of inactivity, especially as we grow older, lead to a decline in the health of our brain. In much the same way as a larger muscle requires more energy to move, a larger brain is also energetically expensive to maintain. The human brain accounts for approximately 20% of the energy an adult burns at rest, which is higher than any other organ relative to its weight (Clarke & Sokoloff, 1999). If we are using it less, then it makes sense that an adaptive evolutionary response is to prune underused structures, reducing the capacity of our brain as an energy-saving measure. As such, age-related atrophy—a decrease in volume in specific regions of our brain that happens as we get older—may, in part, be explained as an energy-saving response to lower amounts of mentally engaging physical activity (Raichlen & Alexander, 2017). But these "use it or lose it" responses to physical and mental inactivity present us with a problem in our modern world. Unlike our early ancestors, we no longer need to run to find food, unless the supermarket is about to close! Our motives for running nowadays are very different from the survival needs of our forebears. So why do we continue to run? What are our motives for running today, when, in all honesty, we simply don't have to?

WHY DO WE CONTINUE TO RUN?

These days we're more likely to dress up as a zebra in a big city marathon than we are to run one into exhaustion across an open savannah. To understand the reasons why many people continue to run today, we first need to understand what motivation is.

WHAT IS MOTIVATION?

Motivation is often vague and hard to define. It is difficult to fully explain why we do something. Motivation can be explained by academics as "the process that influences the initiation, direction, magnitude, perseverance, continuation, and quality of a goal-directed behaviour" (Maehr & Zusho, 2009). But what does this mean in terms of running? The direction of our motivation means what we are trying to achieve. This might be to improve our health, complete a 5k for the first time, or run a personal best time in a marathon. Magnitude refers to the amount of effort we exert to achieve that goal, and perseverance is how long we continue to strive to achieve a goal despite the potential obstacles or setbacks that we might face (Hammer & Podlog, 2016). Some of these ideas are important for running and, as we will explore in Chapter 2, the quantity of motivation, that is, the amount of effort we are willing to exert to achieve a goal, is fundamental to models that attempt to explain the psychological limits of endurance performance.

In addition to the amount of motivation we have, our motives can also differ in terms of quality. One theory that provides an insight into the quality of motivation is called Self-Determination Theory. This theory proposes that our motives can range on a continuum from intrinsic, high-quality motives to extrinsic and lower-quality forms of motivation. We can also experience a complete absence of any motivation for an activity, which is called amotivation (Deci & Ryan, 2000). These types of motivation are what psychologist Lara Mossman refers to as our "flavours of motivation," and each type is shown in Figure 1.1. Assuming we have some motivation to run, then at one end of the continuum are extrinsic motives, which are reasons for running that can be separated from the activity itself. We might be motivated to receive a medal or some other reward, for example, or even to gain the approval of others as a type of social reward. We might also be motivated to run to avoid punishment, such as disapproval from a coach. These types of motivation are considered controlled forms of motivation in that we must act in a specific way to receive a reward or to avoid a punishment. In other words, to receive the medal or gain approval, you might need to finish a race or run a specific time. We might also run to achieve a sense of pride or to avoid feelings of guilt if we skip a run. Again, these are more controlled, extrinsic forms

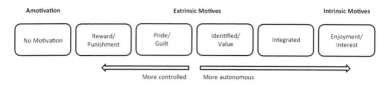

Figure 1.1 The self-determination continuum.

of motivation in that our feelings of guilt or pride are contingent on whether we run or not.

As we move further to the right on Figure 1.1, we begin to find more autonomous or self-controlled forms of motivation. We might run because we identify with and value the benefits that running brings, such as better health or because it lifts our mood, for example. These health benefits include findings that, in comparison with not running, any amount of running, even just once per week, is associated with a lower risk of death from all causes, including heart disease and cancer (Pedisic et al., 2020). Running can also become fully integrated with other parts of our lives and, as a result, we are motivated to run because we see it as part of who we are. In these latter two forms of motivation, running becomes a strong aspect of our identity and, although these are not inherently intrinsic forms of motivation, both value-based and integrated motives are more self-determined and higher-quality forms of motivation than pride/guilt or reward/punishment motives. Finally, at the far right of the continuum are intrinsic motives. Intrinsic motives are those that derive directly from taking part in the activity. These include running because we enjoy it, like the challenge of running, find running interesting, or we are curious to see how far we can push ourselves. These intrinsic motives are the most autonomous, self-determined, and highest-quality forms of motivation.

There are several reasons why it is helpful to understand what motivation is and the different "flavours" of motivation. Each of us can have multiple reasons for running. We might enjoy it, but we can equally value the health benefits it brings or train hard to gain a sense of pride from finishing our first 5k. As such, our motives can incorporate many different flavours. Our primary motives, and the quality of these motives, can also change over time, moving to the left or right of the self-determination continuum. In terms of what keeps us running longer term, research suggests that more autonomous forms of motivation, such a value-based, integrated, or enjoyment/interest reasons, are linked with exercising more and continuing to exercise for a longer term (Teixeira et al., 2012). In other words, enjoying running and valuing what running can bring to our lives are important to maintain longer-term activity. But, as we will later see in Chapter 5, running to avoid feelings of guilt or shame can also be linked with a darker side of running and increase our risk of running addiction.

THE MOTIVATIONS OF RUNNERS

There are also many sources of motivation that are unique to running. Most early research that explored runners' motivations used a scale called the Motivation of Marathoners Scale (MOMS; Masters et al., 1993). You can find the MOMS online at https://sites.google.com/site/motivationsofmarathoners/home if you wish to assess your own motives for running. The MOMS consists of 56 questions and measures a total of nine different motives for running. There are two physical health motives: running for *general health* improvement, such as to improve health or to keep fit, and running because of *weight concerns*, such as to reduce body weight. There are two social motives: *affiliation* with others, such as to meet new people, and receiving *recognition* from others, such as running to earn respect. Two achievement-related motives are *competition* against others and *achieving personal goals*, such as to beat a certain time. Finally, three psychological motives are using running as a *coping strategy*, such as to improve mood or solve problems; running to build *self-esteem*, that is, to build our feelings of value and worth that we have for ourselves; and running to provide a sense of *meaning in life*.

While there are a multitude of reasons for running, many of these motives align with a group of needs called our *basic psychological needs* that, once again, stem from Self-Determination Theory. According to this theory, we each have three basic psychological needs: a need for *autonomy* or a sense of control in our lives, a need for *relatedness* and connection with other people, and a need for *competence* or to feel that we are good at something. Importantly, we are drawn to activities that help to satisfy any one or more of these three needs. Motives to run, such as running for health improvement, to keep fit, to provide greater meaning in life, or using running as a psychological coping strategy, all relate to our psychological need for *autonomy*. Other motives, such as affiliation and recognition, help us feel more connected with others, fulfilling our basic psychological need for *relatedness*. Finally, competing against others and achieving personal goals can give us a sense of *competence* that we are good at running (Zach et al., 2017). What these range of motives highlight is that running can satisfy some psychological needs beyond the basic survival needs of our early ancestors. This helps to explain why humans continue to run today, even though we don't necessarily "have to."

Many studies have used the MOMS to determine which motives drive runners' participation in race events. The first was a study by psychologists Kevin Masters and Benjamin Ogles that explored the motives of 472 recreational marathoners with varying degrees of marathon experience (Masters & Ogles, 1995). They found that the most important reasons for running in rookie marathoners were health-related, such as to improve overall physical health and fitness, and to lose weight. These novices were also motivated to achieve the personal goal of running a marathon and to boost their self-esteem. In turn, mid-level marathoners—those who had previously completed one or two marathons—were mostly motivated to improve their performance, such as breaking a previous best time, and to use running as a strategy to distract from worries and to improve their mood. Finally, the most experienced marathon runners—those who had completed more than three races previously—were primarily motivated by a need for recognition and affiliation with others, for health reasons, and by a desire to compete against others, or what Masters and Ogles termed the "marathon identity." The researchers were surprised by some of the extrinsic motives that existed within this final group, however, such as running for social recognition and affiliation with others, but reasoned that the motive to continue training for multiple marathons requires time and effort—something that may not be possible without the support of family and friends. These more experienced marathoners also grew a social network that involved many other runners, and this social connection provided a source of motivation for experienced marathon runners to continue running. Clearly, multiple motives are important for those who continue to run longer term, and most of us have more than one reason that drives our running activity.

To further highlight these different reasons for running, Masters and Ogles later explored the motives of 1,519 recreational marathoners with best finishing times ranging between 2:15 and 7:04, and identified five broad categories of runners based on the MOMS motives (Ogles & Masters, 2003). These groups were labelled as *running enthusiasts*, those who tend to value running for health, self-esteem, social aspects such as affiliation with others, and achieving personal goals. Second were *lifestyle managers*, those who predominantly ran to improve their physical and psychological wellbeing. Third were *personal goal achievers*, runners who were mainly motivated by their own performance and personal best times. Fourth were *personal accomplishers*, the largest proportion of the marathoners sampled. This group was similar to the lifestyle managers but were more concerned with personal accomplishment and less so about weight management or using running as a psychological coping strategy. The final group were *competitive achievers*, who were more likely than any other group to rate competition with others as a motive for running. The motives and training and demographic characteristics for each group are presented in Table 1.1. Can you recognise your motives and characteristics within any of these running groups?

The motives of runners can also change depending on the event they predominantly participate in. Those that mostly run shorter distances, such as 5km runners, may be less motivated than marathon runners to achieve external recognition, for example (Rozmiarek et al., 2021). In fact, as we will explore in Chapter 6, those who

Table 1.1 Names, motives, and characteristics for marathon running groups.

Group Name	Motives	Characteristics
Running Enthusiasts	Endorse all nine motives for marathoners	Older (40.9 years), mostly female. Previously completed more marathons (9.9 on average). More likely to run with others.
Lifestyle Managers	Personal goal achievement, self-esteem, general health, psychological coping, weight concern, life meaning	Mostly female. More likely to train alone. Complete less training miles and train on fewer days per week. Run slower times.
Personal Goal Achievers	Personal goal achievement	Younger (37.3 years) and mostly male. Faster times (<3 hr 39 min) and complete more training miles (47.3 miles/week) on average.
Personal Accom-plishers	Personal goal achievement, self-esteem, general health	Mostly male. Rated near the middle ("average") on most training characteristics.
Competitive Achievers	Personal goal achievement, self-esteem, general health, competition, life meaning	Younger (35.8 years) and mostly male. Run faster times (<3 hr 28 min). Complete more training days (5.6 days/week) and more likely to train twice a day.

regularly participate in shorter events, such as in weekly 5km parkrun events, often take part to improve their physical and mental health, to meet people, and to have fun. In contrast, ultramarathon runners may be more motivated to participate in their events to provide a sense of meaning in their life, to reach personal goals, and to satisfy a need for achievement. For women ultramarathon runners, improving health and psychological coping are also important motives for running (Krouse et al., 2011). For many ultrarunners, however, trying to beat others is often one of the least important motives for participating in these longer-distance events (Roebuck et al., 2018).

These differences in motivation—our reasons for running—are important and understanding runners' motives can assist coaches or other professionals when they are helping their clients meet their running goals. But sometimes, we get this wrong. When we interviewed an older, beginner 5km runner for a 2020 study (Brick et al., 2020), for example, she told us how her intrinsic motives to enjoy running contrasted with her coach's motives for her to achieve a personal best:

> Even we did a 5 km run . . . and one of our trainers said to me, 'Stop going towards the back, you're going to run it with me!' And I ran it with him, and I did do it quite a lot quicker than normal! . . . And he said, 'See! See!', and I said, 'Yes, but I didn't enjoy it! I hated every minute of that because I pushed myself! If I'd stayed with those ones [slower runners], I'd have enjoyed that run!'

As we will learn in Chapter 4, feeling good when we run and enjoying what we do are important outcomes that help maintain longer-term running activity, especially amongst beginners. Undermining these outcomes can often lead to dropping out from running and other forms of exercise, which is clearly something we want to avoid.

AGE, GENDER, FAMILY STATUS, AND MOTIVATIONS TO RUN

As the preceding quote highlights, older runners, such as those aged 50 years or above, are often more motivated to run for physical health reasons, to provide greater meaning to life, and for social reasons, such as to feel connected with other runners. In contrast, younger runners in their 20s may be more motivated by results or to achieve personal goals (Poczta et al., 2018). These differences can be explained by shifts in our motives as we age and as we gain more experience in running events like marathons. Younger runners may run their first few races to achieve personal goals but, as we age, meeting and connecting with other runners may become more important reasons for continuing to run. Similarly, the many months and years spent training may help more experienced runners notice the mental and physical health benefits they gain from running. While these shifts in motivation mean that our reasons for running can change throughout our lifetime, it doesn't mean that this holds true for everyone. Older runners can be just as motivated to achieve personal goals as their younger counterparts which, once again, highlights how unique and idiosyncratic our motives for running can be (Malchrowicz-Mośko et al., 2020).

Reasons for beginning to run can also differ between male and female runners, with some studies suggesting that males are predominantly motivated by competition or to achieve personal goals, whereas females are more motivated by social reasons, such as taking up running to meet others, to build self-esteem, or to use running as a psychological coping strategy (León-Guereño et al., 2020).

Interestingly, our marital and family status can also influence why we first begin to run or continue running longer term. In one study with marathon runners, beginning to run often resulted from an invitation to take part by a family member or friend, or from viewing running as a convenient form of exercise to improve one's health (Goodsell et al., 2013). Deciding to run a first marathon was also strongly influenced by family members, friends, or running partners. However, unique motives for single, unmarried runners with no children included completing a first marathon to gain a sense of accomplishment, to meet new people, and to accrue some of the physical and mental health benefits associated with running. In contrast, while married runners with no children were also motivated by physical health reasons, they placed more importance on improving their previous best marathon performances and less importance on meeting new people. Interestingly, for this group, running also acted as an emotional-regulation strategy whereby running helped them to manage their emotions and reduce the impact of some emotions on their spouse. Married runners with young children also reported that they frequently used running to form non-family social relationships, to create a separate identity for themselves apart from that as "mum" or "dad," and to provide an emotional outlet outside of family life. Finally, the social relationships that running helped to provide, such as having a running buddy, were important to keep married runners with older children, and those whose children had grown up and left home, involved in the activity.

Taken together, these different motives provide an interesting insight into the many social, physical, and mental health benefits that running can provide depending on our age, experience, and family status. We will explore each of these benefits in much more detail in Chapters 5 and 6.

DOING IT FOR THEM: RUNNING AND ALTRUISTIC MOTIVES

Alongside health-related motives, or those that are focused on satisfying our basic psychological needs, many runners also take part for more altruistic reasons. In a 2008 survey of participants at the Women's Mini-Marathon 10km event in Ireland (see www.vhiwom ensminimarathon.ie/), the largest women's event of its kind in the world, one of the key findings was that over 70% of women cited *raising money for a charity* as their main reason for taking part in the event (Lane et al., 2008). For this reason, while many runners might be considered running enthusiasts or competitive achievers, many others are considered *runners for charity* and are driven to complete running events predominantly for their chosen cause (Nettleton & Hardey, 2006).

Raising money for charity reflects a more altruistic motive that is not immediately tied with our physical health or to our basic psychological needs for autonomy, competence, or relatedness. However, taking part in running events to raise funds or awareness for a charity can encourage people to get more physically active as they train and prepare for the event itself (Bauman et al., 2009). In this way, preparing for and running an event for a charity can lead to many other benefits, such as improved physical and mental health and a growing sense of connection with a charity and with other people. It can also help to build our self-esteem through helping other people and by improving our own physical abilities (Filo et al., 2011). In this way, while many people may be motivated to complete running events for a chosen charity to begin with, there are many additional benefits that accrue by running for such worthy causes.

WHY DO WE QUIT RUNNING?

Although many people maintain their running activity long term, a large proportion also drop out from beginner running programmes within the initial weeks and months after starting. In exercise generally, it is common that 40% to 50% of people will drop out within a couple of months of first taking up a new exercise regimen. Lots of reasons can explain this trend and, for runners, reasons for dropping out include injury, having no previous running experience in their lifetime, and perceiving a lower health-related quality of life (Fokkema et al., 2019). A lack of time and a lack of interest can also explain why some people choose to avoid running events (van Dyck et al., 2017).

Psychologists are also realising that how we feel about running, and how we feel during running, are also important reasons that explain dropout. People who have more negative associations with exercise, such as whether the idea of running immediately fills you with dread or that it is something unpleasant to do, are more likely to drop out of beginner programmes in the early weeks and months (Antoniewicz & Brand, 2016). The opposite is also true, and evaluating running as something "good" or pleasant to do is more likely to lead to better adherence in the longer term. We will explore these ideas, and the importance of feeling good or bad during running, in more detail in the next chapter. Chapters 3 and 4 will build on these ideas further to provide a range of psychological techniques that not only help our running performance, but can also help us stick with running longer term. A key reason for this is that many of these techniques can help to make running feel easier and make it a more pleasant and enjoyable activity to do. Later, in Chapter 6, we will also explore programmes for children and young people that include running, such as The Daily Mile and Girls on the Run. The potential for these programmes to build early, positive experiences associated with running means that we are more likely to evaluate running as something "good" and stick with it into later life as a result.

KEY POINTS ON WHY WE RUN

1. Many features of our body help us to run more efficiently, suggesting a role for running to have shaped our body in our evolutionary past.

2. Running may also have helped to evolve the human brain. Being both physically and mentally active as running hunter-gatherers may have provided a stimulus to shape the structure and function of the human brain.

3. We have many motives for continuing to run today. These include running for health reasons, social reasons, achievement-related reasons, psychological reasons, and altruistic reasons. Our motives can change depending on our age, running experience, gender, and family status.

4. People also drop out from running for many reasons. Some of the most important reasons include how we feel about running and how we feel during running.

5. Understanding why people run, and why people might drop out from running, is important. For coaches, understanding these reasons can help to create an environment where people are more likely to maintain their running activity longer term.

2

WHY DO WE SLOW DOWN OR STOP?

INTRODUCTION

It has long been held that the limits to running performance are physiological. From this perspective, three main factors interact to predict our running performance. These are a runner's maximal oxygen consumption, their lactate threshold, and their running economy (Joyner & Coyle, 2008). Our maximal oxygen consumption (VO_{2max}) is the highest volume of oxygen our body can use, and it sets the upper limit of aerobic metabolism that someone can achieve. It's influenced by the volume of blood our heart can pump, the amount of oxygen our blood can carry, and the capacity of our muscles to extract that oxygen from the blood as it flows though the body. For elite middle-distance and marathon runners, VO_{2max} values in the region of 75 ml/kg/min or higher are often reported (Joyner et al., 2020). Second is our lactate threshold, and it represents the highest fraction of our VO_{2max} that can be sustained during longer-distance running. For elite runners, not only do they tend to have a higher VO_{2max} when compared with lower-level runners, but they are also capable of running for long periods of time at a higher percentage of that VO_{2max}. Well-trained, elite-level marathon runners have lactate threshold values that approach 80–85% of their VO_{2max}. The third factor is running economy and it determines the speed or power that a runner can generate when running at a percentage of their VO_{2max}.

DOI: 10.4324/9781003204206-3

More efficient runners can go faster even when their VO_{2max} and lactate thresholds are equivalent to their competitors.

Alongside these physiological factors, there are also several psychological factors that determine running performance. These psychological factors include motivation, the effort that we perceive, exercise-induced pain, how good or bad we feel (called "affective states" in psychology research), and the strength of our self-belief, or what psychologists call "self-efficacy." Our motives for running, and the quality of different motives, were explored in Chapter 1. In the following sections, we will delve into each of the remaining factors and provide an insight into the effects of these psychological factors on running performance.

PSYCHOLOGICAL FACTORS EXPLAINING RUNNING PERFORMANCE

PERCEIVED EFFORT

Whenever we perform a physical task, like twisting the lid off a jar, lifting weights, or going for a run, we experience a sense of effort. The more we push, whether it is running faster or climbing a steep hill, the harder it feels. We also experience effort when performing mental tasks, such as solving a math puzzle, concentrating intently, or when exerting self-control. Our perception of effort is a mental feeling of work associated with actions like these that provides us with information about the difficulty of whatever task we are performing. If we can acknowledge that something feels easy or hard, then it is because of our ability to sense effort when we perform that task.

In exercise contexts, perception of effort has been studied since the 1960s when Swedish psychologist Gunnar Borg defined perceived exertion as the feeling of how heavy, strenuous, and laborious exercise is (for example, Borg, 1982). Our current definitions are similar, and perceived effort has more recently been defined as the conscious sensation of how hard, heavy, and strenuous a physical task is (Marcora, 2010). To measure perceived effort, participants in running studies are asked questions like, "How hard is it for you to drive your legs and arms and how heavy is your breathing?" Their responses are measured using Rating of Perceived Exertion (RPE) scales developed by Gunnar Borg, one of which is the 15-point RPE scale shown in Figure 2.1. Within this scale, a rating of "6" equates to sitting or lying at rest, whereas a rating of "20" equates to the highest effort you have ever experienced during running. Most runners will rate an easy run at about "9" or "10" on this scale, whereas an intense 800m interval session, or the later stages of a marathon, might feel like a "17" or "18".

Perception of effort plays a crucial role in running and is considered by some as the ultimate factor that limits endurance performance (Marcora & Staiano, 2010). In other words, we slow down or stop during running because of the magnitude of effort that we experience. But perception of effort is malleable, and any factor that increases or decreases perception of effort in highly motivated runners will, in turn, impact how slow or fast they perform.

Rating of Perceived Exertion (RPE)	
6	No Exertion
7	Extremely Light
8	
9	Very Light
10	
11	Light
12	
13	Somewhat Hard
14	
15	Hard
16	
17	Very Hard
18	
19	Extremely Hard
20	Maximal Exertion

Figure 2.1 Borg's 6–20 RPE Scale.

In this book we will present evidence for many psychological interventions that impact perceived effort. Some, such as inducing mental fatigue (see later in this chapter), raise perceptions of effort relative to running intensity and harm running performance as a result. Others, including repeating motivational statements, like "I can do this" (see Chapter 3), have the opposite effect and help us perform better. The key mediator between interventions that harm (such as mental fatigue) or help (such as motivational self-talk) running performance seems to be our perception of effort. Given its importance, perception of effort is central to many models of self-paced endurance performance that we will present in the second half of this chapter.

Although most runners can easily grasp what lower or higher effort feels like, one topic of rich debate amongst endurance researchers is exactly where effort sensations come from. What is understood is that our perception of effort results from the processing of signals in sensory areas of our brain. However, the origin of these signals is less certain. There are two main theories (Pageaux, 2016). First is the *afferent feedback model*, which suggests that perceived effort is generated from the processing of sensory feedback from different parts of our body, including our heart rate, information about lactate production and other metabolic processes in our working muscles, and information about our skin and core temperatures. This is based on evidence of a strong relationship between perceived effort and metabolites produced by working muscles, such as lactate. However, when people are injected with these metabolites at rest (see the next section on *exercise-induced pain*), a procedure that should, according to the afferent feedback model, increase the effort we feel, no such effort is felt. Similarly, when signals returning to the brain from muscles are blocked using epidural-type injections, perception of effort does not decrease as the afferent feedback model would suggest (Bergevin et al., 2023). Together, these findings undermine some of the core proposals of the afferent feedback model.

The second theory is called the *corollary discharge model*, which proposes that our sense of effort results from the processing of a copy of signals that originate from premotor and motor areas of our brain and drive our legs and other muscles to contract during running (including signals from areas of our brain that drive our breathing muscles). Think of this model as hitting the "cc" button on an email. The email (messages to drive your muscles) is sent to the recipient (your muscles), but a copy is also sent elsewhere (in this case, sensory areas of your brain). Your brain interprets the information sent, and you feel this interpretation as a sense of "effort." Consequently, the more your muscles work, through faster running and heavier breathing, the greater your sense of effort. In this model, the key difference from the afferent feedback model is that signals leading to perceived effort originate entirely within our brain. There is much evidence to support the corollary discharge model, with studies showing that our perception of effort can be increased by exercising with fatigued muscles (which need stronger signals from the brain to contract) versus rested muscles, without causing an increase in muscle metabolites, such as lactate (de Morree et al., 2012). Similarly, when we ingest caffeine, our perception of effort is reduced when exercising at the same intensity as without caffeine. Caffeine does not influence muscle metabolites, but it does increase the excitability (or readiness to respond) of nerves in our brain and spinal cord that carry signals to contract toward our working muscles. Because these nerves are more excitable, less activity is needed in motor areas of our brain to stimulate these nerves and our perception of effort seems to be reduced as a result (Cerqueira et al., 2006).

Does this mean that metabolites, such as lactate, play no role in how we feel during running? Well, perhaps not, and the next section will clarify why this is the case.

EXERCISE-INDUCED PAIN

Although effort is an important sensation experienced during endurance performance, we can also distinguish effort from other sensations, such as pain and pleasure (O'Connor & Cook, 1999). Pain is an unpleasant sensory and emotional experience associated with actual or potential tissue damage, such as a strained muscle or sprained ligament. Although we can experience pain from injury, such as a torn hamstring, exercise-induced pain is a separate phenomenon and a natural consequence of running that disappears when we finish a run or slow our pace (Mauger, 2019).

Most of us experience exercise-induced pain as a dull aching or burning sensation in our muscles which is most likely caused by a build-up of metabolic by-products that cause us to experience pain-like sensations. We usually feel this pain during more intense running, such as during 400m maximum pace intervals or during a middle-distance race. Intriguingly, one study tested the theory that exercise-induced pain is caused by metabolic by-products by injecting a solution containing a mix of metabolites produced by working muscles, namely lactate, ATP, and protons (which increase the level of acidity in our muscles during exercise), into the thumb muscles of resting volunteers (Pollak et al., 2014). Injecting a solution that resembled concentrations of these metabolites found at rest produced no pain sensations. However, injecting increasingly stronger mixes that resembled concentrations produced during higher-intensity running provoked stronger pain and fatigue sensations in all participants. The pain was reported as a throbbing "ache" or "hot" sensation in their thumb muscles, similar to the "burning" pain sensations we experience when running. Perhaps even more interesting was the finding that these sensations were only produced when all three metabolites were injected together, providing evidence that exercise-induced pain results from the production of muscle metabolites during higher-intensity activity. This finding also highlights that pain perception is different from effort perception, both in terms of what we feel and the source of these sensations during exercise.

Experiencing exercise-induced pain leads to an urge to reduce or eliminate the pain that we feel. When running, the easiest way to do this is to slow down or stop, because exercise-induced pain is proportional to running intensity. The faster we run, the more painful it can feel. But our experience of pain is also subjective, and while some of us might experience exercise-induced pain as deeply unpleasant, leading to stronger urges to slow or stop, others might experience the same intensity of pain as less of an issue. There can be many reasons for this, including the context (like, "it hurts, but I can see the finish line"), our motivation ("it hurts, but I can win this race!"), and different memories that might change our experience of pain. If you've ever said "never again" after completing a marathon, yet found yourself training for another one six months later, it's likely that your memory of the pain you experienced during the first marathon has been altered in the intervening months by other memories associated with the event, such as the recognition you received afterwards or your motivation to run even faster the next time.

Our training also matters when it comes to managing exercise-induced pain. One difference between trained athletes and non-athletes is that trained individuals are better able to tolerate pain, even though both groups feel pain at a similar threshold (Tesarz et al., 2012). Ultra-distance runners have been shown to tolerate pain induced by dipping their arm in ice-water, known as a cold pressor test, better than non-runners, for example (Freund et al., 2013). There are many reasons for this difference, including better pain-management skills, greater acceptance of pain and embracing it as part of the running experience, and higher beliefs amongst runners that they can deal with pain because of frequent exposure to exercise-induced pain during training and racing. In one study, researchers demonstrated that using unhelpful coping strategies, such as feeling frightened by pain, feeling defeated by pain, and feeling they could not stand their pain anymore, increased runners' odds of quitting during the 2016 RacingThePlanet 250km desert ultramarathon races (Alschuler et al., 2020). In contrast, other researchers have shown that elite endurance athletes use strategies like distraction, relaxation, or motivational self-talk to manage exercise-induced pain more effectively (Lasnier & Durand-Bush, 2022). These strategies, and how you can learn to use them, will be explored in more detail over the next two chapters of this book.

More recent evidence also highlights the importance of the intensity of training to develop higher levels of pain tolerance. In a study led by researchers at Oxford Brookes University in the U.K., 20 healthy adults completed six weeks of either high-intensity interval training (HIIT) or moderate-intensity continuous training on cycle ergometers in a lab (O'Leary et al., 2017). Pain threshold and pain tol-erance were measured before and after the training programme using a test whereby participants performed repeated hand-grip contrac-tions while blood flow to their arm was restricted by a tourniquet—a procedure that induces a burning, pain-like sensation in the arm muscles. Participants also completed two time-to-exhaustion cycling tasks after training ended: one that mirrored a pre-training trial at an intensity that reflected their pre-training fitness levels (called a same *absolute-intensity* trial), and a second trial at an intensity that reflected their post-training fitness improvements (a same *relative-intensity* trial). The results showed that although both groups performed a simi-lar volume of training and had equivalent improvements in fitness levels after training, the HIIT group showed much greater improve-ments in cycling performance. Specifically, the HIIT group improved their performance on the same absolute-intensity trial by 148%, whereas the moderate-intensity group improved by 38%. In the same relative-intensity trial, the HIIT group also improved performance, this time by 43%, whereas performance in the moderate-intensity group was slightly worse. The pain tolerance test produced a sim-ilar finding, with pain tolerance improving by 39% in the HIIT group in comparison with a non-significant 4% improvement in the moderate-intensity group. Across both groups, improvements in pain tolerance were associated with improvements in time to exhaustion in both cycling trials.

Collectively, these studies show that increased pain tolerance con-tributes to improvements in endurance performance independent of changes in fitness levels. Exposing ourselves to exercise-induced pain in training, especially during higher-intensity workouts, and develop-ing mental techniques to manage this pain, are both likely to improve our pain-coping skills and improve running performance as a result.

AFFECTIVE STATES

Like perceived effort and exercise-induced pain, how good or bad we feel during running (an example of what psychologists call "affective states") also has an impact, not only on performance, but also on whether we maintain running longer term. How we feel during running includes feelings of pleasure or displeasure (known as *affective valence*) and feelings of high or low energy (known as *arousal*). In exercise research, affective valence is typically measured using the 11-point Feeling Scale (Hardy & Rejeski, 1989), which asks individuals to rate how good or bad they feel during activity on a scale ranging from +5 ("I feel very good") to -5 ("I feel very bad"). In a similar way, arousal, or how activated and pumped-up we feel, is measured on the six-point Felt Arousal Scale (Svebak & Murgatoyd, 1985), with responses ranging from 1 (low arousal) to 6 (high arousal). These scales are shown in Figure 2.2

How good or bad we feel during exercise is one of the most important factors that determine our levels of physical activity (Ekkekakis et al., 2011). Feeling more pleasure during physical activity is associated higher levels of activity for a longer term. Because of this, anything we can do to feel better during running means we are more likely to stick with it into the future. In Chapters 3 and 4, we will explore some strategies, like listening to music, for example, that can help to make running feel more pleasant and enjoyable. One of the

+5	Very Good	**1 LOW AROUSAL**
+4		
+3	Good	**2**
+2		
+1	Fairly Good	**3**
0	Neutral	
−1	Fairly Bad	**4**
−2		
−3	Bad	**5**
−4		
−5	Very Bad	**6 HIGH AROUSAL**

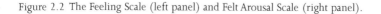

Figure 2.2 The Feeling Scale (left panel) and Felt Arousal Scale (right panel).

biggest factors that changes how we feel during running, however, is the intensity that we go at.

Like perceived effort and exercise-induced pain, how good or bad we feel changes with higher running paces. The critical intensity above which we start to feel worse is known as the *ventilatory threshold*, a point closely related to the lactate threshold and the intensity at which we switch from predominantly aerobic (using oxygen) to predominantly anaerobic (without oxygen) metabolism. When exercising at an intensity below the ventilatory threshold, most people feel good. But as we run at intensities beyond this threshold, we begin to feel worse. You can gauge your own ventilatory threshold by performing a talk test during running. Below your ventilatory threshold intensity, you should be able to speak comfortably and in complete sentences. Above the ventilatory threshold, our ability to speak comfortably is compromised, and we speak in broken sentences or, at the highest intensities, in single words between breaths. If you can speak only a few words before taking a breath and then completing a sentence, you are close to your ventilatory threshold. The pace at which this threshold occurs will depend on many factors, including your levels of training and aerobic fitness.

The key point is that at higher intensities, internal signals from the body, such as our breathing, body temperature, or sensations of effort and exercise-induced pain (collectively known as interoceptive cues), tend to dominate our focus of attention and change how we feel. It's difficult to feel good when our breathing is uncomfortable and we feel high levels of effort and exercise-induced pain. The biggest variability in how we feel happens around the ventilatory threshold. At this point, some people feel good, and some of us feel bad. In turn, the strongest influences on whether we feel good or bad at this intensity are psychological factors, including the strategies we present in Chapters 3 and 4. So, if you want to learn more about feeling better when you run, then those chapters will give you some strategies to put into practice during training and competition.

One other psychological factor that plays an important role in how we feel around the ventilatory threshold is the strength of our belief that we can effectively manage the sensations we feel. This belief is one example of what psychologists call "self-efficacy."

SELF-EFFICACY

Self-efficacy is our belief about what we are capable of doing. More precisely, it is our belief that we can complete the actions needed to produce a specific outcome, and what we know about the importance of self-efficacy comes from the work of Stanford University psychologist Albert Bandura in the late 1970s. Applied to running, if you feel more confident that you can maintain your concentration, perform well in challenging races, manage your thoughts and feelings, deal with bad weather conditions, or pace yourself appropriately, then you have higher self-efficacy beliefs toward running (Anstiss et al., 2018). When these beliefs are higher, we often set more challenging goals, put more effort into a task, and persist through obstacles and difficulties, including a willingness to "suffer" more to achieve the goals we set for ourselves (Bueno et al., 2008). More so, if higher self-efficacy is associated with these positive attributes, then anything we can do to strengthen our self-efficacy beliefs can lead to better running performance. As such, to grow these beliefs, it is important to know where self-efficacy comes from in the first place.

For runners, there are several important sources of self-efficacy beliefs. Recently, researchers at the University of Kent (Anstiss et al., 2020) explored sources of self-efficacy through interviews with 12 endurance athletes, including four distance runners, four triathletes, two cyclists, and two swimmers. They found that the most important source of self-efficacy for these athletes was their *past performance experiences* in both training and competition. These included cumulative experiences, such as successfully completing longer training runs or hitting new personal bests, that strengthened their beliefs over time and provided a reference point for what they could achieve in the future. In other words, when we train and prepare for a race, we're not just getting better physically, we are also building our self-belief about what we are capable of doing in that event. Having persevered through challenges, whether these were difficult moments in races or in life in general, such as a bereavement, also led to an increased belief amongst these athletes in their ability to cope with adversity in the future.

A second source of self-efficacy beliefs for athletes in the University of Kent study were their *physiological states*, including sensations experienced during running, like exercise-induced pain and fatigue, and physical sensations felt in the build-up to an event, such as feeling fit or strong. For these athletes, an awareness of how their body felt influenced their perceptions about what they were capable of achieving in an upcoming race or event. In particular, the athletes reported comparing how they felt at that moment with a knowledge of what they "should" feel like. Any differences, positive or negative, impacted self-efficacy, such that feeling more fatigued than expected in a longer training run lowered it, whereas feeling fitter or stronger than expected increased their self-efficacy.

The third source was *verbal and social persuasion*. This was especially important after a successful experience, such as a strong training run, to reinforce that experience for the athlete. Verbal and social persuasion included support from coaches and training partners and support from family and friends. The words of a trusted coach to provide encouragement or to tell an athlete that they are as well-prepared as they have ever been, for example, was one important source of self-belief, especially when an athlete might have doubted themselves. Linked with this, verbal support also included what runners said to themselves; that is, their "self-talk." The content of runners' self-talk varied depending on the context. For example, during difficult moments in races, self-talk helped athletes push through by reaffirming their ability and recalling past experiences by using statements like "I can push through this. I've gone harder before." Equally, in situations where they doubted themselves, the athletes talked to themselves using motivational or instructional statements to deal with negative thoughts. In Chapter 3 we will explore self-talk in more detail as a psychological strategy that can build our self-efficacy beliefs and improve running performance.

The final source of self-efficacy beliefs were *emotional states*, though these were considered a less important source of self-belief for the athletes. Linked with feelings of anxiety, however, one set of thoughts that were important were doubts and worries. Doubts and worries were highest when athletes were pushing their boundaries and did not have any past successes or similar experiences to draw upon. In turn, those doubts and worries sometimes led to lower self-efficacy beliefs about what they were capable of achieving. But doubts and worries were not always seen as negative or something to avoid. Instead, the majority of athletes felt that their doubts and worries were useful to help them prepare better for an event ahead. Having some doubts kept them "on edge," whereas "being cavalier" meant that they did not prepare as thoroughly as they might. In other words, doubts can be helpful when we use them constructively to optimise our preparation, especially when we have few past experiences to call upon.

Interestingly, which sources of self-efficacy we draw upon to grow our beliefs can also change depending on our level of experience and the stage of a training programme we are at (Samson, 2014). For first-time marathon runners with no previous experience to call upon, the strongest sources of self-belief at the start of a training programme are their physiological states, such as feeling physically in good shape and feeling fit. The next strongest sources are verbal persuasion from others and gaining belief from comparisons with others, including family and friends who might have previously run a marathon. This latter source of self-efficacy is called a *vicarious experience* and, when comparisons are positive, these experiences allow us to believe that "if they can do it, then so can I!" For veteran marathon runners, however, who have a greater array of past experiences to call upon, the strongest sources of self-efficacy at the start of marathon training tend to differ and include their past performance achievements, verbal persuasion (including self-talk), and positive interpretations of their physiological states.

As marathon training progresses, our sources of self-efficacy beliefs also tend to shift. Immediately before the race, the strongest sources of self-belief for beginners are, in order, verbal persuasion from others, how they physically feel, and their performances during training in the build-up to the race. Completing long training runs is an especially important source of self-belief for first-time marathoners. In contrast, for more experienced runners, past performances and verbal persuasion are, once again, their strongest sources of self-efficacy belief immediately before the race. At this point, vicarious experiences seem to be the least important source of self-belief for both beginner and experienced marathon runners. At this point, it's less about what others have done and more about what you feel capable of doing based on your own training, preparation, and past achievements.

Finally, during the race, physiological states, such as feeling energetic or feeling tired and sore, are the most important source of self-efficacy for both beginner and experienced marathon runners, and serve to increase and decrease self-efficacy, respectively. Recalling past training or race experiences, such as getting through tough runs or dealing with poor weather conditions in training, are also important to maintain belief in both groups. Finally, verbal persuasion, both from supporters and runners' own self-talk, are influential during the race. These include family, friends, random people cheering for them along the route, and being able to "tell myself that I can do it."

Collectively, these studies highlight the importance of building self-efficacy beliefs, and the contribution of many different sources to strengthen those beliefs. Improvements in fitness and conditioning as a result of training and preparation appear to be one of the strongest sources of self-efficacy belief for marathon runners (Larumbe-Zabala et al., 2020). But, as this section has shown, other sources are important too. To guide you on how you can intentionally build your self-efficacy beliefs using these sources, at the end of this chapter we will provide an insight into work that we did with an ultramarathon runner to build their self-efficacy beliefs before an extremely challenging ultra-distance event.

MODELS OF SELF-PACED ENDURANCE PERFORMANCE

In the final section of this chapter, we will present some models that have been used to explain endurance performance and, specifically, help us understand what psychological factors impact how fast or slow we run. This section is not intended to be exhaustive, and there are many models that we have not included here. For example, the Central Governor Model (Noakes et al., 2005) is one that many runners might have heard of before. We have not included it here, however, as it has been superseded by a more recent Three-Dimensional Framework of Goal-Directed Exercise Behaviour (Venhorst et al., 2018a), and we will present that model instead. Consequently, in this section we will present two models that are based on the psychological factors explaining endurance performance that are presented in this chapter. These models are The Psychobiological Model (Marcora, 2019) and Venhorst et al.'s (2018) Three-Dimensional Framework.

THE PSYCHOBIOLOGICAL MODEL

The Psychobiological Model, developed by exercise physiologist Samuele Marcora, is based on the principle that endurance performance is a goal-directed behaviour and, as such, performance should ultimately be explainable by psychological factors (Marcora, 2019). Within this model, Marcora includes two psychological constructs that are considered central to explain endurance performance: our perception of effort and our potential motivation. First, Marcora suggests that how we pace ourselves in a running event and how well we ultimately perform is primarily determined by the level of effort we perceive. As a result, according to this model, any physiological (for example, physical training), nutritional (such as caffeine) or psychological manipulation that decreases the perception of effort, and makes a running pace feel easier, will have a positive effect on running performance and allow us to run faster. The opposite is also the case, and any factor that increases the perception of effort will have a detrimental effect on performance.

The second factor, potential motivation, is based on a separate theory called Motivational Intensity Theory (Brehm & Self, 1989). Potential motivation is the maximal amount of effort an individual is willing to exert to succeed on a task. The higher our potential motivation, the more we are willing to exert effort to achieve whatever our goal is, such as finishing a marathon or winning a 5km race. However, this is only true up to a certain point. Once a task is perceived as too difficult, or impossible, then we disengage and, consequently, slow down or quit. Given that perceived effort serves to provide information about the difficulty of a task, the point at which we consciously decide to disengage is determined by the interaction between potential motivation and perceived effort. In other words, the bigger the prize and the more we value that incentive, the higher our potential motivation will be and the greater effort we are willing to exert before we quit.

When it comes to running, three other factors play a role in the decisions we make about how fast or slow to run. In addition to potential motivation and perceived effort, these other factors are our knowledge of the distance we must run (the total distance of a race), knowledge of the distance remaining (how far to go to the finish line), and our previous experience/memory of perceived effort during runs of varying intensity and duration. Most of these factors are self-explanatory. If you run a 5km race and you know that you have completed the first 3kms, then knowledge of the total distance and knowledge of distance remaining are obvious. If this is your first 5km event, however, and you have little experience of racing over any distance, then you may not know how hard you can push over those final 2kms to safely reach the end line. If you are a 5km veteran, then you will know precisely how hard you can push. This "how hard" is determined by our perceived effort and our previous experience plays an important role in pacing events correctly. Recently, we (Brick et al., 2019) added to these factors by highlighting that knowledge of the difficulty of the remaining distance, that is, whether it is flat or contains a steep incline, for example, also impacts a runner's pace-related decision-making. The more challenging we think the remaining distance will be, the more conservatively we tend to pace our run.

A THREE-DIMENSIONAL FRAMEWORK OF GOAL-DIRECTED EXERCISE BEHAVIOUR

More recently, sports physician and exercise scientist Andreas Venhorst and colleagues proposed a three-dimensional framework to understand pacing and performance in endurance activities, like running (Venhorst et al., 2018a). They argued that previous models, like Marcora's Psychobiological Model, rely exclusively on ratings of perceived effort, and that other psychological factors are equally important to explain endurance performance.

There are three main dimensions within this framework. The first dimension is *perceived strain*, or perceived effort, which Venhorst and colleagues suggest can be split into perceived physical strain or the strength of the physical sensations coming from our legs, lungs, and body in terms of "light" or "strong," and perceived mental strain, or the perceived difficulty of a task in terms of "easy" or "hard." Both physical strain and mental strain can be measured separately using ratings of perceived effort scales. The second dimension is *core affect*, which is split into affective valence (how good or bad we feel) and arousal (how pumped up we feel). We explained both of these factors earlier in the affective states section. The third dimension is *mindset*, which comprises both flow states and action crises. A flow state involves complete absorption in an activity, where running feels almost effortless and enjoyable, and where the challenge of a running task is matched by our ability to perform it. An action crisis, however, is when we experience a conflict between continuing to run and slowing or quitting—the type of overwhelming experience many runners encounter when they "hit the wall" in the latter stages of a marathon and leads to strong urges to slow down or stop.

The three-dimensional framework makes several predictions. First, it suggests that perceived mental strain and perceived physical strain are the primary regulators of how fast or slow we run. The easier a run feels, the faster we are likely to go. This is similar to the predictions of Marcora's Psychobiological Model. Second, core affect is also important, and feeling bad or having lower energy also negatively impacts running performance. Finally, experiencing an action crisis during running results in a mindset shift that influences decisions we make about persisting or slowing/quitting during a run.

Some evidence for this model exists. During competitive, head-to-head cycling over 70km, Venhorst and colleagues showed that falling behind an opponent led cyclists to feel worse (lower affective valence) and to the development of an action crisis whereby the cyclists experienced strong urges to give up the chase (Venhorst et al., 2018b). Interestingly, when comparing a head-to-head trial versus an individual trial in this study, winners felt better when they were ahead of an opponent in comparison with how they felt at the same distance during a solo ride, whereas losers felt worse after falling behind and experienced a stronger stress response as a result. In turn, falling behind and feeling worse led to an action crisis amongst losers that ultimately resulted in reduced commitment to the task and a slower performance in comparison with their solo ride.

The framework has also been tested with runners by asking highly trained individuals to complete three 20km treadmill time-trials: once as a familiarisation trial, once in a rested state, and once in a fatigued state after completing a series of 100 drop-jumps from a 45cm height before the run (Venhorst et al., 2018c). The fatigue induced by the drop-jump intervention mimicked the sensations a runner might experience in their legs toward the later stages of a marathon or ultra-marathon. The drop-jumps and subsequent fatigue meant that runners experienced greater feelings of strain in their body (physical strain) that led them to feel worse (lower valence) and, consequently, experience a larger action crisis during the fatigued 20km trial than the rested one. Ultimately, the runners completed the 20km time-trial approximately 4% slower in the fatigued stated than when rested.

Both Marcora's Psychobiological Model and Venhorst et al.'s Three-Dimensional Framework provide an insight into psychological factors that influence running performance. They suggest that motivation, perceived effort, affective states, and mindset are all important variables that determine our running performance. Different factors can influence each of these states, including how we perform relative to an opponent, or the muscle damage and physical fatigue that accumulates during prolonged running. The psychological techniques we use during training and races, such as our self-talk, the goals we set, or how we appraise a situation, can also influence these psychological factors, and these techniques will be the focus of Chapter 3. One further factor that can also have a detrimental effect on running performance, however, is the level of mental fatigue that we experience.

"I'M TIRED!" MENTAL FATIGUE AND RUNNING PERFORMANCE

Mental fatigue results when we engage in prolonged periods of demanding mental activity. It might accrue from a long day of work or when we experience disrupted sleep. When mentally fatigued, we feel tired, a lack of energy, lower alertness, and, unless we are highly motivated, our ability to perform mental tasks is compromised. An intriguing question that endurance researchers have explored is whether mental fatigue also impacts endurance performance. One reason is that endurance tasks, like self-paced running, require us to control our thoughts, emotions, and actions (Van Cutsem et al., 2017). In other words, to run well we must overcome negative thoughts, stay focused, deal with unpleasant sensations and high levels of effort, and make decisions about whether to maintain our current pace, speed up, or slow down. Running well requires intense concentration and an ability to override urges to slow or stop, and our ability to perform these mental challenges may be compromised when mentally fatigued.

In experiments, mental fatigue is often induced by asking participants to engage in a prolonged cognitive task, such as performing a task called the Stroop Colour-Word Task. A demo of the Stroop task can be found by exploring the library of experiments at www.psytoolkit.org/. The Stroop task involves a number of cognitive functions, including sustained attention and working memory. Participants are presented with a colour word on a screen (for instance, blue), that is written either in a congruent (in this example, blue) or incongruent (for example, green) coloured font. Participants must respond by selecting the font colour rather than the colour word, which is especially challenging in the incongruent condition. So, in this example, if the word "blue" is written in green font, then "green" is the correct response. One of the key features of the incongruent tasks is response inhibition, where we must override our automatic response (such as to select "blue") in favour of the correct response (selecting "green"). Intense running has a similar requirement, where we must override strong urges to slow down or stop in order to maintain a goal pace or to finish a race. Given that both tasks require similar cognitive functions, fatigue caused by one should have a knock-on, negative impact on the second.

Several studies have shown the impact of mental fatigue on endurance performance. In the first experimental study, Samuele Marcora and colleagues showed that participants performed worse on a time-to-exhaustion cycling trial when mentally fatigued (lasting 640 seconds) versus when rested (lasting 754 seconds) (Marcora et al., 2009). Importantly, mental fatigue had no effect on any physiological variable, including heart rate or levels of blood lactate, meaning that these variables had no impact on cycling performance between trials. Participants' motivation to give their best effort was also unaffected by mental fatigue. However, mental fatigue did impact the ratings of perceived effort such that the mentally fatigued cycling trial felt harder than the rested trial. Based on these findings, the authors concluded that endurance performance is ultimately limited by psychological factors, such as perceived effort, rather than physiological factors, like blood lactate or heart rate. Their findings provided evidence to support some of the key assumptions of Marcora's Psychobiological Model.

Short-duration mental tasks, such as completing 10 minutes of the Stroop task, do not seem to impact running performance. This is probably because shorter tasks are not mentally fatiguing. However, when we do mentally taxing work for a longer period of time, such as performing difficult mental tasks for at least 30 minutes, then our running performance can suffer. In one study, for example, performance on a 5km treadmill run was more than one minute slower when mentally fatigued (completed in 24.4 minutes) than when mentally rested (23.1 minutes) (Pageaux et al., 2014). Similarly, mental fatigue following 90 minutes of a concentration task impacted 3km running times on an indoor track such that participants, once again, ran slower when mentally fatigued (completed in 12:12 mins) than when mentally rested (11:58 mins) (MacMahon et al., 2014). In both studies, participants reported that both runs felt equally hard, despite running slower in the mentally fatigued condition. This once again shows that mental fatigue raises our perceptions of effort relative to our running pace. Outside of controlled experimental settings, mental fatigue may also impact running performance in real-world events, with mentally fatigued runners in one study completing a half-marathon event four minutes slower on average than participants who read magazines and were mentally rested before the race (Gattoni et al., 2021). This time difference was not statistically significant, however, leaving some doubt about the true impact of mental fatigue on running performance in real-world conditions.

Interestingly, our ability to resist mental fatigue might be improved with longer-term physical training. In one study, performing 30 minutes of the Stroop task had no effect on the cycling performance of professional cyclists in comparison with a rested trial, whereas the performance of recreational cyclists was worse after engaging in the same 30-minute task (Martin et al., 2016). This might be because a high level of training enabled the professional cyclists to ward off the effects of the 30-minute task and allowed them to tolerate a greater amount of mental exertion without experiencing mental fatigue and, consequently, without impacting their cycling performance. Physical training, then, might not only improve our physical resilience, but also increase our ability to resist the detrimental effects of mental fatigue on running performance.

Although there seems to be some strong evidence that mental fatigue can impact endurance performance, how mental fatigue exerts this impact is not completely understood. The effects are not physical; neither heart rate, muscle metabolism, nor muscle function are impacted by mental fatigue (Martin et al., 2018). Mental fatigue does impact perceived effort, however, and perceived effort is higher, or the speed produced at the same level of perceived effort is slower, when performing in a mentally fatigued state compared with a rested state. One mechanism to potentially explain the effects of mental fatigue on running performance is an increase in a substance called *adenosine* in regions of our brain. Adenosine accumulates in our brain during waking hours and dissipates when we sleep. It is one reason why we feel mentally tired at the end of a long day or when our sleep is disrupted. Adenosine also accumulates in our brain during effortful mental activity. One important region of the brain affected by adenosine accumulation is the anterior cingulate cortex, a region involved in tasks that require effortful self-control and is linked with perseverance, processing of emotions, performance monitoring, and perceived effort during endurance tasks. As such, accumulation of adenosine can impact running performance in several ways by increasing perceived effort and by lowering our ability to exert self-control and persist during effortful tasks (Martin et al., 2018). As such, avoiding mental fatigue, or doing something to minimise its impact (like ingesting caffeine), is an important pre-event strategy to help optimise your running performance.

KEY POINTS ON WHY WE SLOW DOWN

1. There are many physiological and psychological factors that determine how well we run. Each are important, but the ultimate limits to running performance may be psychological.

2. Psychological factors that determine running performance include motivation, perceived effort, exercise-induced pain, how good or bad we feel (affective valence), and self-efficacy beliefs. Any manipulation that changes these factors can have a positive or negative impact on running performance.

3. Key models of endurance performance, including the Psychobiological Model and the Three-Dimensional Framework of Goal-Directed

Exercise Behaviour, provide an insight into how these psychological factors interact to determine running performance.

4. Psychological strategies can have a positive effect on running performance and improve running adherence. They can do so by lowering perceived effort and exercise-induced pain, increasing how good we feel during running, and strengthening our self-efficacy beliefs. We will explore these psychological strategies in the next two chapters.

5. Mental fatigue can have a detrimental impact on running performance. Avoiding mentally fatiguing activities before races is important to help you perform at your best.

RUN WITH IT: HOW CAN I BUILD MY SELF-EFFICACY BELIEFS?

Self-efficacy—our beliefs about what we are capable of achieving—is something that we have worked to develop and build with a lot of runners. One example is that of "Chris." Chris was already a very competent runner when we first started to work together, with personal bests of 16:50 minutes in the 5km, over 10 miles in 61:33 minutes, and 82:59 minutes over the half-marathon distance. But when we first started to work with Chris, he was preparing for a new challenge and was in training for the 250km Spartathlon event in Greece (www.spartathlon.gr/en). Chris had never run over this distance before and, without any past performance experiences, he was feeling daunted by the prospect of what lay ahead and whether he could successfully complete the event.

To qualify for the Spartathlon, certain entry criteria must be fulfilled, including the challenging task of completing a race of at least 120km (men) or 110km distance (women) within a 12-hour limit in the previous two years. Chris completed a qualifying race in the months before our first meeting and, having achieved the criterion and qualified for the Spartathlon, one of the main mental challenges for Chris was the thought of running for somewhere in the region of 35 to 36 hours during the race. To add to the challenge, Chris didn't just want to finish the event, but also wished to race it competitively and finish in 35 hours. Because of this, we needed to develop Chris's belief that not only could he finish the event, but also his belief that he could be competitive and "race" the event.

Our work with Chris began nine months before the Spartathlon and focused on drawing from key sources of self-efficacy beliefs for runners, including *past-performance experiences*, interpretation of *physiological states* and *emotional states*, *vicarious experiences*, and *verbal and social persuasion*, including support from his family. One of the first sources of self-efficacy that we drew on was Chris's past performance experiences from his training, preparation, and race events. Chris had a good level of self-belief in his abilities as a runner, and this came from the times he had achieved over shorter events. His performance in the 120km qualifying event also gave him a stronger belief that he could compete over longer distances. However, to build upon these successes, Chris wanted to achieve new personal bests over shorter race distances in preparation for the Spartathlon. This included running his first sub-3-hour marathon—something that most previous 35-hour Spartathlon finishers from the U.K. had achieved. After reaching this milestone, Chris reflected that, "Knowing that other 35-hour runners of similar standard had also achieved this goal gave me the motivation and incentive that I could do it too!" (A *performance achievement* combined with a *vicarious experience*.)

We reflected that those successful performances, like his first sub-3-hour marathon, came from meticulous training and preparation, and reframed the doubts and anxiety (*emotional states*) that Chris had about the event as useful thoughts that would help ensure he prepared as well as he possibly could be. This preparation included physical training, like running and strength training, and other important aspects, like optimising his nutrition and hydration plans for the Spartathlon. We also asked Chris to keep a training diary to maintain a record of his training and preparation throughout the build-up to the Spartathlon and to note any milestone achievements, such as a new personal best or a new longest run. This ensured that his self-efficacy was not based on one particular event or success, but instead was accumulated across all aspects of his training, preparation, and racing in the months leading up to the event.

Chris also had to manage other challenges in his life during these nine months. While he was dedicated to training and preparation, he also had a one-year-old child and had recently started a new business with his dad. While this made finding the time to train properly, eat well, and get sufficient sleep a challenge, Chris felt that if he could juggle those commitments and persevere through difficult moments in his working-life, he could draw on those experiences to manage difficult moments during the race itself. In this way, the challenges became a positive that built his belief that he could cope with challenges during the race. The stress of a sleepless night with a young child—something that Chris initially worried would hinder his preparation—was reframed as a positive as it allowed him to occasionally train in a mentally fatigued state, for example—something that he would undoubtedly experience in the 35-hour Spartathlon race, too.

One challenge that Chris was not sure he could deal with was his ability to cope with running in hot conditions. Temperatures during the Spartathlon event often exceed 30°C, whereas Chris was more familiar with cooler temperatures in the U.K. To help prepare for these conditions, Chris undertook 90-minute sessions of Bikram hot yoga in the middle of 22-mile-long training runs to mimic the intense heat he would experience during the Spartathlon event. This helped Chris to replicate, to a certain extent, some of the physiological states he might experience in Greece, including feeling warm and experiencing strong thirst sensations. This also allowed Chris to practice his hydration plans for the race, and ensure that he drank sufficiently to avoid extreme dehydration. Finally, training in a dehydrated and often fatigued state, but working to maintain a target race pace, made Chris more aware of the negative thoughts and urges to slow down or stop that he experienced. We worked with Chris to develop a self-talk plan to counter these urges and negative thoughts. This self-talk plan included reminders of all the challenges and difficulties that Chris had faced in training and previous races, and how he overcame these. We developed and practiced simple statements that focused on building self-efficacy beliefs, like, "I've gone harder and felt worse in training, I can do this too." More importantly, by pushing himself in training, Chris developed new experiences of overcoming adversity that he could draw on during the race. In this way, difficult training sessions became a key focus, as they provided opportunities to practice and refine his self-talk strategies for the race itself. Ultimately, this preparation proved important in the Spartathlon race when Chris was running alone, without the support of others around him, and needed to talk himself through these lonely miles to stay positive and focused on the task at hand.

As a final source of self-efficacy belief, we reflected that Chris could not do all of this by himself. He was supported in the whole venture by his wife, who moved some of her work shifts to care for their child and accommodate his training runs, for example. Chris reflected that she was his biggest cheerleader at races and other events, and this support added to his beliefs that he could prepare for and achieve his goals in the Spartathlon. Further, his dad and brother would crew for him in the main event, providing nutrition and hydration support, alongside encouragement that would help him maintain his beliefs through some difficult moments in the race that he expected to encounter.

During the event, Chris drew on each of the sources of self-efficacy beliefs that we worked on during the nine months of preparation. One of the most important sources came during the toughest moments of the race when he drew on support from his family. Chris had a picture of his son on his backpack that he would look at during brief stops at race checkpoints. He later reflected that "It meant the world to me to give everything to the race and try and demonstrate a legacy for my son." Having his wife and son at the finish line provided additional motivation to get to the finish and to push through difficult parts of the race. Chris ultimately finished the Spartathlon in under 35 hours (his main performance goal) and finished in the top 150 places for the event.

3

WHAT WILL HELP ME RUN FASTER?

INTRODUCTION

Psychological interventions aim to improve running performance by manipulating one or more of the psychological factors that we explored in Chapter 2. These interventions can help lower the effort we perceive, manage exercise-induced pain, improve affective states, or build our self-efficacy beliefs. By doing so, they can improve our running performance. But before we delve deeper into these psychological interventions, it is useful to begin by clarifying some terms that we will use in this chapter.

In sport and exercise psychology, we can differentiate between psychological skills, psychological techniques (or psychological strategies; we will use these terms interchangeably), and psychological interventions (Birrer & Morgan, 2010). Psychological skills can help us cope with the psychological demands of running, including a need to stay motivated over long periods of training (motivational skills), to manage effort or deal with exercise-induced pain (volitional skills), or to stay focused and avoid distractions during a competitive race (attentional skills). Each of these psychological skills can, in turn, be developed with training in the use of psychological techniques. These techniques, such as goal setting and motivational self-talk, will be the focus of this chapter. Finally, a psychological intervention might be developed by a sport and exercise psychologist to include training

DOI: 10.4324/9781003204206-4

in one or more psychological techniques with the end goal often being to improve running performance and/or to increase running enjoyment.

This chapter will provide you with insight into psychological techniques that can improve each of the psychological skills important to running performance. To help you learn and apply these techniques, at the end of this chapter we will provide an example of an intervention with one runner we worked with to help them achieve their goal of running a marathon in a personal best time. Given this, goal setting seems a logical technique to begin this chapter with.

GOAL SETTING

SETTING SPECIFIC GOALS

Most runners set goals of some sort. Often, these goals are focussed on the *outcome* of an event, like winning a race or on reaching a specific level of *performance*, like achieving a new personal best time. We can also set *process goals*; that is, goals that are focused on implementing specific strategies or actions, such as speaking to ourselves in an encouraging way during difficult moments in a race (Filby et al., 1999). We will discuss these processes in more depth as we go through this chapter. What we know for sporting performers, however, is that both process goals and performance goals significantly help to improve performance and increase our beliefs about what we are capable of achieving. More so, the biggest improvements in performance and self-efficacy beliefs come from setting, and focusing on, process goals, whereas performance goals can lead us to try harder, feel more confident, and lower symptoms of pre-performance anxiety (Williamson et al., 2022). Outcome goals do not seem to have these beneficial effects.

In terms of performance goal setting, the conventional wisdom according to goal-setting theory is that setting specific and difficult goals helps to focus our attention on the task at hand, increases our effort and persistence, and ultimately leads to short- and long-term performance gains (Locke & Latham, 1985). The more difficult the goal is, the more it increases our effort and persistence and, ultimately, leads to greater performance gains than easy or "do your best" goals.

While these principles of goal setting are relatively easy to understand, whether they improve running performance as goal-setting theory predicts is less clear. One study, for example, found that a four-week goal-setting intervention in which the researchers set what they considered easy (improve your time by 5%), difficult but realistic (improve by 10%), and unattainable (improve by 15%) performance goals resulted in similar levels of improvement amongst a group of 28 female high school runners over a 2.3km distance (Tenenbaum et al., 1999). Interestingly, despite what the researchers considered in terms of goal difficulty, the runners themselves did not always perceive their goals in the same way. Some in the easy goal group perceived their goal as very difficult, for example, whereas some in the realistic goal group felt that their target was easy. These perceptions might have impacted the runners' beliefs about whether they could achieve their goals by the end of the four-week period, ultimately impacting the effort they exerted to train for, and achieve, their goal.

An intriguing study with Boston Marathon qualifiers supports this point—that what matters is how difficult we perceive a goal to be. Qualifying for the Boston Marathon means running faster than a specific time based on your age and gender. As runners move into older age categories, the qualifying standards get progressively slower to accommodate age-related reductions in performance. When researchers analysed the data of 145,544 qualifiers between 1970 and 2015 (Burdina et al., 2017), they found that runners who went up an age category—specifically those who moved into the 45–49 and 50–54 age groups, and thus had a challenging, yet more attainable goal to aim for—performed better in qualifying than younger runners who remained in the same age category. In contrast, much older runners whose qualifying standards got a lot easier—such as those moving into the 60–64 age group and beyond—demonstrated a relative drop in their performance levels.

The implications from these studies are important. Performance goals we perceive as too easy are not very motivating. Consequently, we tend to exert less effort to pursue them. We don't prepare as well as we might, and our subsequent performance can suffer. In contrast, goals that we perceive as too difficult can be demotivating, lowering our belief that we can reach them, which often means that we give up prematurely (Kyllo & Landers, 1995). Not only that, trying to achieve goals that we consider too hard can increase performance-related anxiety and lower our level of performance as a result (Lane et al., 1995). Specific performance goals that we perceive as challenging, moderately difficult, and attainable motivate us to try harder and persist for longer in our attempts to achieve them.

So how can we use these insights to help us perform better during running events? One application is to allow for some goal flexibility when it comes to race day, especially when conditions like warm temperatures or high winds can change how achievable we consider our goal. One strategy is to set different levels of performance goals, which might include a best-case, *dream goal*; a *happy goal* for less-than-ideal conditions; and an *acceptable goal* for worst-case scenarios (Meijen et al., 2017). Having different levels to our goals, and being flexible with how we apply them, can help us stay motivated, maintain our beliefs about what we can achieve, and reduce anxiety when race day comes.

SETTING OPEN GOALS

Specific goals aren't the only types of goals that we can set. Recently, researchers have explored the effects of non-specific goals, including one type of non-specific goal called *open goals*. Open goals differ from specific goals insofar as while specific performance goals provide a fixed target, open goals are exploratory and instead focus on "seeing how far I can go" or "seeing how fast I can run." Some recent studies have explored the effects of open goals on exercise tasks. In a 2020 study, for example, 78 healthy adults were asked to complete three six-minute walks (Swann et al., 2020). After a first walk to determine each person's distance achieved, the study participants were randomly assigned to different groups with either a specific performance goal (asked to walk 16.67% further during the second walk and 8.33% further during the third walk), an open goal (instructed to see how far they could walk in six minutes during walks two and three), a do-your-best goal (asked to do their best for six minutes), or no goal (asked to walk at their normal pace).

Perhaps not surprisingly, the findings revealed that the three "goal" groups walked further than the no-goal group in walks two and three. What was surprising, however, was that the three goal groups did not differ in the total distance walked between each other. There were important differences in terms of how each group felt, however. Those who were given specific performance goals reported feeling higher tension and more pressure to achieve their target during each walk. In contrast, those given open goals reported higher perceptions of their performance than the other goal groups despite no difference in actual performance between each group. In a follow-up study, people who were considered inactive before the study walked further during the six-minute period and, despite walking further, reported feeling better and enjoyed their walk more when they set an open goal in comparison with a specific goal. In contrast, previously active individuals achieved greater distances and reported greater enjoyment when they set a specific goal in comparison with an open goal (Hawkins et al., 2020).

What these studies suggest is that specific performance goals can make us feel pressured to achieve a fixed target. This is not necessarily a bad thing, and this pressure can motivate experienced walkers or runners to achieve higher performance levels. But, for beginners, especially if the priority is to get more active or to enjoy a walk or run and to feel better during it, then setting an open goal, such as to start running and "see how far I can go" or "see how well I can do," might be a better strategy to employ.

More recently, in a study led by University of Lincoln researcher Patricia Jackman (Jackman et al., 2021), we've found that setting non-specific goals, like open goals, flexible performance goals, or even do-your-best goals, were more likely to help induce flow during running—a pleasant and enjoyable "in the zone" high-performance state where running feels effortless and comfortable. In contrast, setting specific performance goals were more likely to lead to a clutch state—one where runners still performed at their best, but running felt hard and required the use of a multitude of psychological strategies to reach the performance level they were striving for. In other words, these runners were working hard mentally to reach high performance levels and the strategies used included motivational self-talk, imagery, and chunking. Each of these strategies are presented in the following sections of this chapter and it is to the latter strategy, chunking, that we will turn our attention to next.

CHUNKING

One way to mentally deal with the challenge of longer distance events, like a marathon, ultramarathon, or even your first 5km, is to mentally break it down into smaller, more manageable chunks. This strategy is called chunking, and it is a technique that runners at all levels use to get through races that, otherwise, might seem overwhelming. In one of our interview studies (Brick et al., 2015), an Olympic marathoner revealed how she broke the distance down in her own mind from the start of the race:

> You cannot stand at the start line of a marathon and go, 'I am going to run 26.2 miles today.' You'd go insane! So I break it into really small chunks. I break it into five-mile chunks, and I think, 'How will I feel when I get to 10 miles?' Especially in a [13.1-mile] half marathon, I have this point at eight miles where I say to myself, 'I'm nearly at 10.'

We've also found that beginner runners learn a similar strategy. One beginner runner from a later study (Brick et al., 2020) reported how she used chunking during a 5km race to overcome urges to stop and ultimately make it to the finish line:

In my own head, the last 5k that I did . . . it was just lamppost to lamppost, and it was like, 'Right, I can see something', and I focused on a car . . . that was parked . . . and once I got to that car, I focused on to the next thing I could see.

Why is chunking a strategy that so many runners find helpful? In many ways, chunking involves a process called *attentional narrowing*, whereby individuals focus their attention directly on a nearby object, like a lamppost just ahead, rather than letting their eyes move around and explore the surrounding environment more broadly. Researchers have found that when people use attentional narrowing, they estimate that the focused-on object, a lamppost or a tree, for example, seems closer than it appears when focusing on the wider surroundings (Cole et al., 2014). In other words, how far we feel we have left to go to reach our imaginary finish line is less when we narrow our attention toward that object and focus on getting to it.

In studies exploring the effect of attentional narrowing, people have been found to walk faster and be more physically active in a typical week, including walking and running more, when narrowing their attention onto interesting objects in their environment and focusing on reaching them (Balcetis et al., 2020). There are different reasons that might help to explain this phenomenon. Narrowing our attention on something just ahead can help us stay focused, strengthen our belief that we will reach that imaginary finish line, and convince us that achieving our goal is closer than it might otherwise be. In turn, we might be more motivated to work harder, and run faster, to get there and to experience some satisfaction when we do. Chunking a bigger distance like a marathon in this way, and mentally hopping from one imaginary finish line to the next, makes a hard task seem easier and more manageable, and gives us mini targets to achieve as we progress toward the finish. As one participant in a recent study we completed put it, "I was using little goals along the way. There were points along the route where I was saying to myself, 'if you get to this point, then that's a win'" (Jackman et al., 2021). This example also shows how chunking can be combined with our next strategy, self-talk, to further help running performance.

SELF-TALK

Self-talk includes all those statements that we say to ourselves either silently in our heads or out loud. Some of that self-talk is spontaneous and, when it comes to running faster, our spontaneous self-talk can often be unhelpful. How many times have you caught yourself in the middle of a hard run repeating statements like, "This feels awful," "I can't do this," or "I can't go any further"? But our self-talk can also be directed toward goals we are trying to achieve. So, we might say, "Get to the finish line" or, if using a chunking strategy, "if you get to the next turn, then that's a win."

What sport psychology researchers have found is that our self-talk has a big impact on how we feel and how we perform during running by helping us deal with high levels of effort and exercise-induced pain. There are many different types of self-talk. We might talk to ourselves to guide our pacing ("Stick to a 5 minutes per kilometre pace"), to build our self-efficacy beliefs ("You've prepared well; all that training is in the tank"), or to manage our emotions and stay calm before a race ("Take a deep breath and relax"). Two types of self-talk that have received the most attention in running research, however, are motivational self-talk and instructional self-talk. Instructional self-talk is often used to direct our focus (for example, "focus on the vest of the runner ahead") or to guide our actions (for example, "pump your arms"), and we will learn more about the benefits of these cues in Chapter 4. Motivational self-talk includes statements like, "Come on, keep going" or "Keep pushing," and research has shown that repeating these statements can increase self-efficacy, lower perceived effort, and optimise our pace. In endurance activities like running or cycling, training people to strategically use motivational self-talk statements has been shown to increase the length of time people can keep going at a fixed intensity before stopping (Blanchfield et al., 2014), improve 10km cycling performance times (Barwood et al., 2015), and enhance performance in hot conditions (Hatzigeorgiadis et al., 2018).

In one study with runners, 110 marathoners were split into two groups (Schüler & Langens, 2007). Half of the runners received training in self-talk and statements focused on self-encouragement, such as "stay on; don't give up"; anticipation of positive outcomes, such as "I will be proud of myself if I can do it"; and self-calming instructions, such as "stay calm and you will do it." The researchers were interested to know how these statements helped runners deal with an *action crisis*—a phenomenon we introduced in Chapter 2 as overwhelming thoughts about stopping or quitting, and something that marathon runners often experience at about 20 miles into the race. The researchers found that although both groups of runners experienced similar thoughts about stopping or quitting, the runners trained in self-talk were better able to overcome their action crises and held a better pace over the last six miles of the race. In other words, when needed, having self-talk strategies to call on helped the runners through their crisis moments and they achieved a higher level of performance as a result.

Self-talk can also help runners in other distances, ranging from 800m to ultra-marathon. In a study with three experienced 800m runners, for example, learning to use self-talk statements such as reminders to run "smooth and fast" (an example of instructional self-talk) or "you got this" (motivational self-talk) helped to improve their 800m performance times by between 8% (17 seconds) and 9.8% (25 seconds), while also delaying the urge to slow down (Cooper et al., 2021). With ultra-runners, a self-talk training intervention failed to show any effects on running performance in a 60-mile event with participants in a no-intervention control group completing the event in a similar time to a group trained in self-talk (McCormick et al., 2018). Despite this, however, runners in the self-talk group found the intervention helpful and continued to use it six months after the study had ended. That latter finding was positive, but this study highlights one of the research challenges in this field. Most studies tend to take place in controlled laboratory environments, and studies such as this—exploring the effects of a psychological intervention in race situations—are extremely challenging to complete. But we need more of these studies to demonstrate the benefits (or not) of psychological strategies like self-talk in real-world settings.

More recent studies have also revealed that *how* we speak to ourselves can be as important as what we say to ourselves. In one study, researchers found that speaking to ourselves in the second person (for instance, "you can do this") versus in the first person (for instance, "I can do this") helped to improve cycling performance, with participants cycling 2.2% faster over a 10km time-trial when using second-person versus first-person statements (Hardy et al., 2019). Despite their faster pace, the cycling task felt no harder when participants spoke to themselves using the second person ("you . . .") statements. In a similar way, framing an effortful endurance task as a challenge, but one that we can overcome (for instance, "this is tough, but I can push through it") can also be helpful. When compared with the negative statements that we often repeat to ourselves when activities feel hard, for example, "my legs are tired," challenge-focused self-talk statements have been shown to improve performance during 20 minutes of constant-pace cycling, with participants cycling 200m further when repeating challenge-focused statements to themselves in comparison with negative statements (DeWolfe et al., 2021). What these studies show is that the content of our self-talk is important and that learning, developing, and strategically using self-talk can help to improve running performance (Latinjak et al., 2019).

RELAXATION STRATEGIES

Runners can also learn and use several different relaxation techniques to help their performance. One relaxation technique is called progressive muscle relaxation (PMR). PMR is a sophisticated technique that requires some training to perfect but has been shown to help lower anxiety and relieve tension in everyday life (McCallie et al., 2006). PMR involves tensing and relaxing each of our muscle groups in a sequence that begins with the hands and ends with the feet.

The purpose of the PMR technique to become more aware of tension in our muscles and, when we notice it, to be able to release that tension and relax. The entire PMR sequence takes about 15 minutes to complete, and you can find audio scripts for PMR online through a quick search for "progressive muscle relaxation."

A second technique is centering breathing. Centering involves taking a slow, deep breath and pushing your belly out as you breathe in to completely fill your lungs. When you breathe in, you become aware of the of tension in your body and let that tension go on the breath out with a slow, strong exhalation. A single centering breath should take approximately 10 seconds, with breathing in lasting for a count of four or five seconds, and slowly breathing out for a count of five or six seconds. The purpose is to control your arousal levels, relax if needed, and focus your attention on the task at hand.

Most studies with runners have looked at the effects of these relaxation strategies on running economy; that is, how efficient an athlete is as measured by the amount of oxygen used when running at a specific pace. As introduced in Chapter 2, running economy is a physiological factor that determines running performance and the more efficient we are the faster we can potentially run. Running economy is measured in a laboratory where specialised equipment is used to determine the oxygen used and carbon dioxide produced when running. While many factors can influence running economy, including the shoes that we wear, economical runners also focus more on staying relaxed during running, even when feeling pain or fatigue during a race (Smith et al., 1995). This can take some time to master, but the ability to stay relaxed can be trained and improved in less economical runners using the relaxation techniques outlined in this section. In one study, a six-week relaxation training intervention consisting of PMR and centering breathing resulted in a large improvement in running economy and a lower heart rate when running at lactate threshold intensity—a comfortably hard pace for most runners (Caird et al., 1999).

More recently, we (Brick et al., 2018) noted a small improvement in running economy following a brief-contact intervention to smile when running in comparison with both frowning and a usual focus (control) condition. No such improvements were noted for an active relaxation condition where participants were instructed to consciously relax their hands and upper body when running. In contrast, when participants were frowning—that is, mimicking a facial expression associated with intense effort—perception of effort was higher than when smiling and when focusing on relaxing their hands and upper body. Whether this works for all individuals is unknown, however, as not all runners in our study benefitted from smiling. Clearly, more research is needed into the effects of these strategies on longer-term running performance.

Collectively, what these studies show is that benefiting from a relaxation technique like PMR or learning to relax during running takes some practice and time to perfect. But there are some additional benefits to these strategies beyond improvements in running economy. Learning how to manage our pre-race anxiety by using deep breathing can help us to stay calm and focused, for example (Stanley et al., 2012). This can also have an impact on our pacing strategy, with one study showing that runners who used deep breathing to lower feelings of anxiety or anger reported higher calmness and had a more even pacing strategy during 1600m running (four laps around a track) than runners who increased the intensity of these emotions or those who used no strategies to control these emotions (Lane et al., 2016a). In this way, relaxation can help us avoid situations where we go out too fast at the start of a race, for example—a mistake often made by more anxious or less-experienced runners, and one that can often have catastrophic consequences for our overall performance.

MENTAL IMAGERY

Imagery is a mental experience that mimics a real-life experience. When we use mental imagery, we often experience many of the sensations associated with the real experience, such as seeing and feeling our movements or hearing sounds associated with the real experience. Mental imagery differs from dreams in that when we use mental imagery, we are awake and conscious, and we often perform mental imagery for a specific purpose. These purposes might be to mentally practice a skill or technique, to rehearse a tactical plan or strategy, to imagine dealing with the emotions that accompany performance, or to imagine successfully dealing with difficult situations during competition. In this way, we can use mental imagery as a technique to improve psychological skills like motivation, attention, or volitional skills to deal with the effort, discomfort, or pain associated with running performance.

Few studies have explored the effects of imagery training alone on running performance. Imagery has been used as one part of a package of mental techniques used with runners, however, and we will present an insight into those studies later in this chapter. Of the studies focused on imagery alone, one had a group of non-athlete college students use mental imagery over 12 weeks in one of four conditions: either to imagine perfect running skill execution, to imagine successful performance outcomes to build motivation, to imagine a combination of both, and a no-imagery group that received lectures instead (Burhans et al., 1988). Running performance was measured every four weeks over a 1.5-mile race. After the first four weeks, the running-skills imagery group showed greater improvement in performance relative to the lecture-only group, but no differences between groups were evidence at end of the 12 weeks, suggesting that mental imagery focused on perfect skill execution or motivational imagery might have short-term benefits, but may not be a useful long-term psychological strategy to improve running performance.

Interestingly, some studies have also explored how imagery can help change how we feel when completing endurance tasks. We know from Chapter 2 that feeling good or feeling bad during running is important for longer-term adherence. Over two separate studies, researchers from the University of Birmingham asked participants to complete 20 minutes of moderate-intensity cycling while imagining a time they found exercise either enjoyable or energising. For runners, this might be a run during which you felt great, enjoyed good company or pleasant scenery, or a time when running fast felt effortless. Using these types of imagery, the researchers in the University of Birmingham study found that vivid enjoyment-focused or energy-focused imagery helped participants feel better and more revitalised both during and after activity than when using no imagery or when imagining cycling with good technique. Using any type of imagery also helped make the cycling task feel more enjoyable than no imagery (Stanley & Cumming, 2010a, 2010b). Combining both enjoyment- and energy-focused imagery at moderate intensities also helps to shift our focus from unpleasant bodily sensations during activity and, by doing so, make exercise feel more pleasant in comparison with using no imagery (Tempest & Parfitt, 2013). In this way, using imagery can help make running feel better and more enjoyable, potentially increasing both performance and longer-term running activity as a result.

REAPPRAISAL

Reappraisal involves changing what we think about a situation or the meaning we give to it. So, for example, when out for a training run, I might turn a corner and find myself running into a headwind. If I immediately start to think, "I hate headwinds! I never run well into a headwind," then I will probably feel some negative emotions as a result, like feeling tense, frustrated, or annoyed. But if I reframe that same headwind as an opportunity to practice some psychological strategies, like a challenge-focused self-talk statement ("Yes, this headwind is tough, but you can push through it"), staying relaxed, or chunking the distance ("Just get to the next lamppost"), then I might feel a different set of emotions, like feeling calmer or feeling excited to see how well my strategies work. If I notice that I navigated the headwind in a much better way than usual, I might also feel proud of how I dealt with a usually tricky situation. As this example highlights, by changing the meaning we give to a situation, reappraisal helps to change the emotions we subsequently feel and often leads to more positive and less negative emotional states.

One study has explored the effects of reappraisal on running performance (Giles et al., 2018). The researchers asked 24 trained runners to complete three 90-minute treadmill runs at a moderate intensity (heart rate between 75% and 85% of maximum) on three separate days, each one week apart. For the first run, the runners received no special instructions. On the second and third runs, however, they were asked to either reappraise how they felt or to distract themselves from how they felt. For reappraisal, the runners were instructed to think of the running experience objectively and analytically and adopt an emotionless attitude, like a scientist would. In other words, they were asked to think more rationally about their running experience. In the distraction run, the runners were asked to focus on anything emotionally neutral (such as buildings on the university campus) instead of their running experience and how they were feeling.

The findings revealed that when using the reappraisal strategy the runners reported that the 90-minute run felt easier and that they felt less "worked-up" (that is, lower levels of arousal) than during the no-instructions run, despite no differences in how far they ran or in their heart rate between these two runs. There were no differences between reappraisal and distraction in terms how easy the run felt, or how good or bad they felt during the run, however. This suggests that changing what we think about our experiences during running can help change how we feel, and that reappraisal can be another tool in our box of techniques to help lower perceived effort, optimise our running experiences, and potentially improve running performance.

MULTI-MODAL PSYCHOLOGICAL INTERVENTION PACKAGES

Although it is useful to understand how single psychological techniques, like relaxation or motivational self-talk, help our performance as runners, in reality we often use multiple techniques rather than just one alone when performing at our best. We might set moderately difficult performance goals, focus on staying relaxed, and talk ourselves through challenging moments. In line with this approach, some studies have explored the effects of a package of more than one psychological technique on running performance. These packages include a combination of goal setting, self-talk, relaxation, or imagery, and most have shown beneficial effects on performance. More so, many of the mental techniques seem to work better in combination. Imagery, for example, can be used to mentally rehearse staying relaxed, or to practice using motivational statements to get through difficult moments in a race.

In one study, a group of four athletes were trained in a package of techniques that included setting daily and long-term performance and outcome goals, inducing relaxation via PMR and centering breathing, developing positive and motivational self-talk statements, and using imagery to plan for competition-specific scenarios. The effect of the psychological-skills training intervention on running performance was tested using a series of 1600m runs and the findings revealed that the runners improved their average 1600m time by between eight seconds and 29 seconds over the duration of the intervention (Patrick & Hrycaiko, 1998).

Combinations of these techniques also helped performance in a simulated triathlon event, where participants completed a 2km row, a 5km cycle, and a 3km treadmill run either by themselves (Thelwell & Greenlees, 2001) or in a head-to-head competition (Thelwell & Greenlees, 2003). Intriguingly, the competitive triathlons provided a deeper insight into how participants used each of the mental techniques to help their performance. For goal setting, participants used a combination of outcome (for example, to win), performance (for example, achieve a time for each element of the triathlon), and process (for example, use self-talk during the competition to go faster) goals. In combination, while outcome goals helped to build motivation, process goals gave athletes a specific focus for each section of the race which, in turn, helped to build confidence. Relaxation strategies, like PMR and centering breathing, were used pre-race to help get into the right "zone." During the race, relaxation also helped participants focus on their process goals, get their pacing strategy right, and deal with the higher effort they felt during the final running section. Imagery helped most during the running phase, where participants tried to imagine themselves being relaxed to stay focused on their process goals and to deal with the effort they felt. In addition, one participant imagined running on a track to mentally chunk the 3km treadmill run into shorter, more manageable segments. Finally, self-talk was used to stay motivated and manage the effort they felt during the run, and to maintain good running technique (for example, "upright stance") when the final phase felt hard.

Some mental techniques are also more helpful than others, depending on the conditions. When running in hot (30° Celsius) conditions, for example, a group of participants ran 1.15km (8%) further during a 90-minute treadmill run after receiving training in psychological techniques compared with before this training (Barwood et al., 2008). Like other studies in this area, the post-training run did not feel any harder than the previous run despite a faster speed, emphasising that these psychological strategies can help to lower the effort we perceive. When preparing to run in the hot conditions, the runners also reported that mental imagery (imagining overcoming the fatigue they would feel at different points in the run) and performance goals (targeting running 5% to 10% further in the final run) were the most useful. During the run, using mental imagery (imagining being behind or ahead of a competitor to increase motivation); using challenge-focused statements, such as, "this is a challenge I'm going to meet, I have the mental tools to cope," or instructions, such as, "head up, shoulders back, and keep my stride length"; and focusing on process goals (mentally breaking the 90-minute run into smaller 15- or 30-minute chunks) were reported as most useful to help performance, whereas centering breathing to relax was rated as the least useful. What these studies highlight is that having a range of psychological strategies at your disposal is beneficial to running performance, but some can be more useful than others, depending on the context you find yourself in.

MENTAL CONTRASTING WITH IF-THEN PLANNING

What Chapter 2 and the present chapter have highlighted is that many of the challenges associated with running can be predicted.

We can predict—even if you've never ran one before—that running a marathon will feel hard toward the latter stages. You might also expect hills or a headwind at some point along a race route. If you are competitive, you might expect to be ahead in a race or struggling behind a competitor. Each of these scenarios bring psychological challenges that we need to respond to in the best possible way. In some cases, like research on self-talk has shown, using motivational statements can help us through crisis moments. As such, what's often more important is not the events that happen to us, but how we respond to them. One strategy that can help us to respond better in challenging situations is "if-then" planning.

If-then planning—or implementation intentions (Gollwitzer, 1999)—is a strategy whereby we first identify potential obstacles or challenges that can impact our performance. These are the "ifs." How we would like to respond to these challenges, or what will help to maintain our performance, are the "thens," and these responses can be planned as part of our pre-race preparation.

Some studies have explored the effects of if-then planning with runners. In one study, if-then planning helped participants change the intensity of specific emotions, like increase how happy and energetic they felt, by using an if-plan, such as, "If I wish to feel more energetic, then I will focus on positive emotions that help me run." Although, the if-then planning group were no more effective than a goal-setting group or no-intervention control group at regulating these emotions (Lane et al., 2016b). Meijen et al. (2021) asked participants in their study to consider four potential stressors or challenges that they might encounter during an upcoming race (that is, "ifs") and think of potential strategies for dealing with each challenge (that is, "thens"). Examples of strategies included focusing on their breathing or encouraging themselves to relax. After formulating their if-then plans, participants were encouraged to practice and refine them in the build-up to their race. The findings revealed that people who developed if-then plans perceived that they had more control over the stressors they encountered during their races than a no-intervention control group, even though both groups rated the stressors they encountered as equally intense. In other sports, such as tennis, if-then planning has also helped players to increase concentration and effort and deal with unhelpful thoughts and feelings by implementing a range of coping responses, such as remaining calm or using positive self-talk. As a result, players trained in the use of if-then planning rated their performance in a critical match as better in comparison with a group of players who received no such training (Achtziger et al., 2008).

These studies highlight some useful ways that if-then planning can help runners regulate their emotions, cope with stressful and challenging situations, increase concentration, or deal with unhelpful thoughts. Using the strategies presented in this chapter, you can practice using if-then planning to help with challenging aspects of running. Applying research on goal setting and relaxation, for example, a marathon runner might avoid going too fast at the start of a race ("if") by focusing on staying relaxed and implementing a process goal to run at a specific pace. Similarly, if experiencing an urge to slow down or stop during a race, then you might plan to repeat some motivational statements to help maintain your running pace. If running up a steep hill, then you might plan to narrow your attention and chunk the distance, focusing on getting to the nearest landmark, and then repeat, until the hill is scaled.

Sometimes, however, it can be difficult to know exactly what the best course of action is to take at a particular moment. For example, if it is tough during a race and you are experiencing a crisis moment, should you persist with your "dream" goal or adjust your pace to achieve your "happy" goal? One additional strategy that can help in this regard is called mental contrasting (Oettingen, 2012). Mental contrasting is a problem-solving technique whereby we first imagine a future goal or wish, and also imagine the best possible outcome, like finishing a race in a new personal best time or beating a competitor. Next, we contrast that outcome with our present reality, like what our current pace is, how far we have left to go, or how hard the challenge will be. Mental contrasting helps us realise the actions we need to take if we are to progress from where we are now, overcome potential obstacles, and get to where we want to be. It can also help us weigh whether persisting with a goal or changing it is the best course of action to take.

Combining mental contrasting with if-then planning can be an effective strategy for runners and has been shown to reduce the number of obstacles people perceive when trying to achieve a goal. In other words, by having considered the challenge and developing a plan to overcome potential hurdles along the way, then we perceive fewer obstacles to achieving our goal because we have an effective plan that helps us overcome obstacles more efficiently (Riddell et al., 2023). Together, this process can be summarised in four steps—*Wish, Outcome, Obstacle*, and *Plan* (WOOP)—that can lead to better performance in many areas of life, including changing health-related behaviours like exercising more and eating fewer unhealthy snacks. You can learn more about this process at www.woopmylife.org.

In a recent study, we (Jackman et al., in press) interviewed runners who reported having an optimal experience during a race. This including winning a race, setting a world record, or running a personal best. We found that these runners often reported using mental contrasting and if-then planning during races to help them deal with challenging situations. The strategy also helped them decide whether their pre-race goals were realistic in the moment and to adapt these goals if needed. One half-marathon runner reported using mental contrasting, if-then planning, and a combination of other psychological techniques like motivational self-talk to help with decision-making, accept the pain they would experience, and persist with their pre-race goal during a critical moment in the race:

> You are always worried in the middle of a race that the wheels could come off, that you could run out of energy, or something happens and you just slow down. You are always worried about that, but you are going, 'let's deal with this pace, let's keep going'. You just keep taking it a bit at a time. I wouldn't really break it into miles or anything like that, I just keep going, 'yeah I feel okay', and then in another bit, 'yeah I feel okay', and in the last

two miles, I am going, 'I am going to have to dig deep now and, even to hold the same pace I have been doing, I am going to have to hurt a bit more'.

What this example shows is that mental contrasting, if-then planning, and having a range of psychological techniques to call on in the moment can be effective to help runners perform at their best despite the challenges they face during a race.

KEY POINTS ON PSYCHOLOGICAL STRATEGIES DURING RUNNING

1. Specific goals that are challenging, moderately difficult, but also attainable motivate us to try harder and persist for longer in our attempts to achieve them. Specific goals are linked with better performance in more experienced athletes.
2. Non-specific goals, such as open goals that say "see how well I can do," can help beginner runners to perform better, feel better, feel less tension and pressure, and enjoy running more than specific goals. Open goals can also help us experience flow during running.
3. Mentally breaking a task down—chunking—helps running performance by increasing focus, making difficult tasks seem more manageable, and building our belief that we can achieve a performance or outcome goal.
4. Motivational self-talk can help runners deal with high levels of effort and improve running performance. Experiment with what you say to yourself (for example, "I can do this") and how you say it (for example, "You can do this"), and find what statements work best for you.
5. Relaxation techniques can help to improve running economy. They can also help us stay calm and focused before races, manage sensations of effort, and help us stick to a pre-planned race pace.
6. Energy- or enjoyment-focused mental imagery can help us feel better during moderate-intensity running by shifting our focus away from unpleasant bodily sensations.

7. Reappraisal, or changing what we think about our running experiences, such as thinking more rationally about the physical sensations we experience, can help to make running feel easier.

8. If-then planning can help us prepare for challenging situations and respond to them in the best possible way. Combining this with mental contrasting can help us make better decisions about pacing and actions we need to take to perform at our best during races.

RUN WITH IT: HOW CAN I USE PSYCHOLOGICAL STRATEGIES TO HELP ME RUN FASTER?

The strategies presented in this chapter can be helpful for runners at any level who want to improve their performance. To give you an example of how these can be applied, we worked with Russell, a 29-year-old U.K.-based elite-level runner who completed his first marathon in under 2 hours and 20 minutes. After this performance, his new goals were to represent his country internationally, but he recognised some areas he needed to work on to improve his overall performance. These areas included dealing better with pre-race anxiety, which he felt impacted his overall performance in his last marathon, and managing the effort and discomfort he experienced during the final six miles of the marathon, something he did not deal with well in this first marathon, and he felt that he lost a lot of time as a result.

Over six sessions in the 12-week build-up to his next marathon, we worked on several psychological strategies with Russell. Our initial discussions focused on goal setting. Russell's original goals for the marathon, developed alongside his coach, were outcome and performance-based. His outcome goal was to place within the top five runners from his country, a result that would qualify him to compete internationally. His performance goal was to set a new personal best time somewhere between 2 hours 10 minutes and 2 hours 15 minutes. In our first session, we discussed these goals and, although we didn't change these goals, we worked toward shifting Russell toward more controllable, process-oriented goals to focus on during the race. This would help his focus during the race and help reduce his pre-performance anxiety stemming from an excessive focus on less-controllable outcomes. We discussed what would help Russell achieve his outcome and performance goals, and together we developed three areas to work on:

- To have a plan to deal with the effort and physical discomfort he would experience during the latter stages of the race and maintain his goal pace to the finish line.
- To stick to the pacing strategy agreed upon with his coach pre-race. In his last marathon, Russell's pre-race anxiety meant that he abandoned his pre-race plan and went too fast at the start.
- To stay focused throughout the race.

To help achieve each of these processes, we introduced Russell to several psychological strategies that he could use during the marathon. First was self-talk that he could use to deal with the effort and discomfort experienced during the later stages of the race. We developed some statements in our second session that Russell then refined during long training runs and tough interval sessions in the build-up to the marathon. The key was to keep these statements short, memorable, and focused on what he wanted to achieve. Some examples of motivational statements that Russell found worked well for him included, "How bad do you want it?", "Dig deeper," "This pain is just a thought," and "Be more Fauble!" (Scott Fauble is an American marathon runner and Russell admired his ability to push himself through tough training and races). We also developed some instructional statements to help Russell focus on specific actions and to optimise his pace when he began to struggle during the race. Examples of these statements were, "Drive your arms!", "Concentrate!", and "Keep relaxed."

To help Russell stay focused on key processes during each stage of the race, we introduced Russell to chunking and encouraged him to develop this strategy in training. Russell practiced chunking by mentally breaking his longer training runs into 5km segments. Each 5km had a specific focus, such as "staying in the moment" and keeping to the pacing plan over the first 5km. Russell achieved this by thinking of "standing up tall, staying relaxed, swinging his arms, and having a nice stride and turnover" during this segment.

More intense training runs also helped to mimic the latter stages of a marathon and the fatigue he might feel. For example, one long-run training session included a 20km segment performed at a pace faster than his goal marathon pace and was exceptionally challenging to complete. When Russell encountered difficult patches and experienced anxiety or negative thoughts during this session, instead of "panicking" as he previously might have, we encouraged him to reappraise these sensations as a normal and a welcome sign that he was digging deep. His plan was to respond to these feelings by guiding his focus back to his running cadence, rhythm, and self-talk strategy to "dig deeper." After this training run, Russell reflected that, although the idea of embracing discomfort was new to him, it helped him to refocus and have a strategy to deal with the sensations he experienced. Finally, after each 5km segment was completed in training, Russell would take a sip of an energy drink to "reward" his efforts before focusing on the next 5km segment to come.

In the immediate build-up to the marathon, we introduced Russell to some additional strategies to help his pre-race focus and deal with pre-race anxiety. First was mental imagery. Russell combined imagery training with music and later recounted:

> I did imagery every day for the two weeks before the race in the taper. I had a playlist of 3 songs that would get me in the zone each day. I then imagined difficult situations in the race that I would have to overcome. I then listened to the same playlist on race morning to get me in the zone and to bring back those memories of successfully overcoming difficult patches in training to help build my confidence on race morning.

We combined mental imagery training with if-then planning in the pre-race build-up, and a key focus was to plan responses for "what if" obstacles, like "What if I get a stitch in the last 6 miles?" His planned responses, such as, "to stay calm and take deep breaths," could be called on, if required, to stay calm, focused, and have practical strategies to implement if they were needed. In the six weeks before the marathon, Russell trialled these techniques in a half-marathon event and subsequently strengthened his belief in this approach to race planning based on how effective he felt his planned responses were in that race.

Russell ultimately achieved his performance goal, completing the marathon in under 2 hours and 15 minutes. He also finished in his country's top five finishers, achieving his outcome goal. Russell later reflected that his pre-race planning gave him confidence on the start line, knowing that he had a plan in mind should difficulties arise. In the race, he felt calmer through harder parts as he felt he had "been there before," which helped him overcome difficult moments and stay on pace to achieve his goals. He also reflected that practicing the various strategies, such as deep breathing, self-talk statements, and chunking in training helped them come to mind more "naturally" during the race and were easier to implement as a result. He also reflected that:

> I thought I had a few moments of flow, but mostly it felt really hard, and I was utilising the techniques throughout the duration of the race. We left no stone unturned. I felt more confident and calmer on the start line than I'd ever done before.

4

WHAT SHOULD I FOCUS MY ATTENTION ON?

INTRODUCTION

Attention refers to our ability to focus on objects, thoughts, feelings, or actions. For runners, this might mean focusing on a lamppost just ahead, the feelings of effort that come from running fast, or reminding yourself to run with relaxed hands and arms. Our attention allows us to focus on the task at hand, ignore distractions, and to stay alert for the duration of a race, and it can be directed in one of two ways. Sometimes we intentionally focus on certain things, like mentally latching on to the vest of the runner in front of you and doing everything you can to stay as close as possible to them. At other times, our attention can be captured by something unexpected or important. You might suddenly become aware of a competitor's footsteps drawing closer from behind, your breathing might be so hard that it's difficult to ignore, or you get distracted by a scenic view along a new running route.

As runners, what we focus on impacts on many aspects of performance and our running experience. Our focus of attention can help us run faster. It can also make running feel easier or harder or make running a more pleasant or unpleasant activity to do. In this chapter, we will provide an overview of research on the effects of attentional focus on running outcomes. This will begin with a brief overview of

DOI: 10.4324/9781003204206-5

what attentional focus is and how we categorise the various things that runners focus on. We will then explore the effects of attentional strategies on running performance, on perceived effort (that is, how easy or hard a run feels) and on affective responses during running (that is, how good or bad we feel). This chapter will also consider the effects of specific strategies, such as music and mindfulness, on running performance and on how we feel during running.

WHAT DO RUNNERS FOCUS ON?

One of the first studies to explore what runners pay attention to separated our focus into two broad categories, *association* and *dissociation* (Morgan & Pollock, 1977). In their work, researchers William Morgan and Michael Pollock interviewed 19 world-class long-distance runners, including eight marathon runners with performance times better than 2 hours 20 minutes for the distance. To perform at that level, Morgan and Pollock anticipated that these runners had some way of distracting themselves from the effort and pain they might experience during a race. To their surprise, however, they found that instead of distracting themselves from these sensations, these runners used an *associative* strategy. That is, they tuned in and paid close attention to physical sensations, like their breathing or how their muscles felt, while they ran. Although these runners wore a watch when running, they mostly paced themselves by "reading their bodies," and periodically reminded themselves to relax and stay loose as they ran.

The association strategy of these elite runners differed from that of lower-level marathoners. Morgan and Pollock found that slower runners, those who completed the marathon in three to four hours, tended to *dissociate* from bodily sensations during races. Although these runners thought a lot when they ran, very rarely did these thoughts turn to the act of running. Instead, they distracted or tuned away from these sensations by thinking about past experiences in their lives, performing mental puzzles, imagining listening to music, or singing songs to themselves. One of the most memorable distraction techniques from one runner was "stepping on the imaginary faces of two co-workers she detests throughout the marathon"! Based on these findings, Morgan and Pollock suggested that what runners focus on is a simple case of either association or dissociation, and that elite runners tune in to how they feel and pace accordingly, whereas lower-level runners tune out and distract themselves throughout a run.

Despite its simplicity, the association/dissociation model oversimplifies the attentional focus of runners. Instead, most peoples' attention shifts toward multiple sources of information throughout a run. A runner might switch their focus from attending to how they feel to optimising their running technique, staying relaxed, or on various distractions they encounter as they run. A runner's thoughts during a training run will also differ from those in a race, regardless of their level of ability (Masters & Ogles, 1998). Similarly, running at a higher intensity or on a challenging route feels harder, and the bodily sensations that result, such as heavier breathing or activity-induced muscle pain, tend to capture and dominate our focus of attention. Each of these nuances highlights that a runner's focus of attention is variable, flexible, and dynamic, shifting according the demands of different situations (Lind et al., 2009). As a result, how we think about attentional focus needs to reflect the dynamic nature of our attention when we run.

Since Morgan and Pollock's work, other researchers developed more refined ways of categorising runners' attentional focus. South African psychologist Helgo Schomer, for example, explored the mental strategies of marathoners (Schomer, 1986). Schomer asked runners to wear a voice recorder and to speak aloud anything that came to mind while they ran. Based on the recordings, Schomer developed ten separate categories of thoughts, including focusing on task-related thoughts like *body monitoring* (such as breathing, painful muscles), *pace monitoring*, or issuing *commands and instructions* to themselves, such as "relax your shoulders" or "go easy." The runners also focused on task-unrelated thoughts, such as *personal problem-solving*, *reflective thoughts*, or focusing on their *work or career*. Based on these ideas, Schomer (1987) developed a mental-strategy training programme that helped marathon runners distinguish between task-related, associative thoughts and task-unrelated, distracting thoughts. The purpose of the programme was to help runners focus on more task-related thoughts as they ran and to optimise their running performance as a consequence.

A decade after Schomer's work, Stevinson and Biddle (1998) explored how our thoughts can lead to "hitting the wall"—the point in marathon running, typically at about 20 miles, where a runner's pace drops significantly due to a depletion of muscle glycogen stores, low blood glucose, and running-induced muscle damage. In their study, Stevinson and Biddle developed a 2 X 2 classification system, suggesting that associative thoughts can be classified as either *inward monitoring* (for example, focusing on bodily sensations during running, such as our breathing, muscle soreness, thirst, or sweating) or *outward monitoring* (for example, focusing on things important to running performance, such as split times, the running route, mile markers, or water stations). Similarly, dissociative thoughts can be classified as either *inward distraction* (for example, focusing on irrelevant thoughts such a daydreaming, imagining music, or solving math puzzles) or *outward distraction* (focusing outwardly on things unimportant to the running task, such as on the scenery or spectators). When analysing the thoughts of runners who reported "hitting the wall" versus those who didn't, Stevinson and Biddle (1998) noted that those who hit the wall reported more inward distraction, such as daydreaming, earlier in the race. In other words, those who hit the wall paid less attention to how they felt or on reading their body as they ran, tended to run too fast earlier in the race as a result, and these pacing errors had negative consequences for their performance later in the race. This finding provides some important clues about attentional focus and optimal running performance that we'll discuss later in this chapter.

More recently, we (Brick et al., 2014) reviewed 112 studies on the effects of attentional focus on endurance activity. Based on the research evidence, we expanded on Stevinson and Biddle's model to suggest that inward monitoring can be further divided into a focus on monitoring bodily sensations (*internal sensory monitoring*) and efforts to control our thoughts, feelings, or actions (we called this *active self-regulation*). We also suggested that distractive thoughts can either be active or involuntary. In other words, sometimes we choose to deliberately distract ourselves, whereas at other times our attention is captured by external objects or our own thoughts.

In the next sections, we will provide some insights on the effects of different attentional focus strategies and how we can apply these insights to help our own running experiences. We will begin with the evidence on associative, task-related thoughts and how these can help us run faster and perform better. Later, we'll turn our attention to distractive thoughts and answer a separate question: How can our focus of attention help make running a more pleasant and enjoyable experience?

FOCUS: TUNING IN AND RUNNING PERFORMANCE

When we first start to run, bodily sensations like heavy breathing or exercise-induced pain tend to dominate our focus of attention. It's not that we focus on these sensations intentionally. Instead, it's that the volume is so loud that our focus is captured by these sensations and we are unable focus on much else. As a result, these sensations often make running an unpleasant experience. For one beginner runner that we interviewed for a 2020 study (Brick et al., 2020), her focus on breathing led to some negative thoughts about running. She recounted her early running experiences as:

> I couldn't get my breathing right at the start. My total attention was on breathing . . . it took me weeks to regulate it! And it was only once I had that, that I was able to focus on anything else. It was totally just on being able to do my breathing and, 'Why am I doing this, why am I putting myself through it? I hate this, I hate running! Why am I doing it?'

The good news for beginner runners is that these sensations get easier to manage as our fitness improves. However, the quote highlights an important point. When we focus excessively on bodily sensations, not only does running feel harder and less pleasant, but our performance can also be slower as a result. As such, learning how to deal with these physical sensations is one of the first mental challenges that a runner faces. Anything we can do to shift our focus away from these sensations will help us perform better and help make running a more pleasant experience.

In terms of running performance, this does not mean that we should ignore these sensations completely. As shown in the Stevinson and Biddle (1998) study, marathon runners who distracted too much from these sensations tended to make pacing mistakes that led to hitting the wall later in the race. Instead, what's more helpful is to tune in to these sensations periodically. That is, check in and perform a body scan now and again during a run and use these bodily sensations as a source of information to adjust your pacing, if necessary. In the same study with beginner runners (Brick et al., 2020), a second runner explained how, with experience, they learned to read their body and to use these sensations as a source of information to help with pace-related decision-making:

> That has been the big factor . . . I know whenever I'm starting off now, I'm not busting myself and I know after a couple of miles I'm not going to be exhausted . . . Before it was an unknown how I was going to feel after a mile . . . Now I'm taking it easy and if I feel . . . better . . . I go a bit faster. But if I know I'm going too fast, I'll slow down again. And I'm always thinking, 'How do I feel? . . . Is my breathing heavy?' And if all that's ok, I can go!

To highlight the importance of tuning in to running performance, a study led by psychologist Rick LaCaille had 60 experienced runners complete three five-kilometre runs (LaCaille et al., 2004). One run took place on a 200-meter indoor running track, one on a flat outdoor road route, and one on an indoor treadmill. During each run, half the runners were asked to pay attention to the heart rate and pace readings on their watch every 30 seconds. This was an association-type strategy. The remaining runners distracted themselves from the running task by listening to music as they ran.

Regardless of their strategy, all of the runners were instructed to run as fast as they liked during each run. Following each run, participants rated how hard each run felt.

The findings revealed that runners who tuned in to their heart rate and pacing ran, on average, 1 minute and 47 seconds faster than the musically distracted group over the 5km runs. Monitoring pace and heart rate helped runners to perform at a level that was more consistent with their abilities and improved performance times as a result. In line with our earlier recommendations, the authors concluded that *periodically* monitoring bodily sensations and tuning in to a pace consistent with one's abilities allows for better performance when running faster is a priority.

Interestingly, running on the treadmill was significantly slower, by about four minutes, than both the outdoor and track 5km runs. Despite this slower pace, running on the treadmill felt *harder* than both of the other runs. This finding emphasises our other key point about focusing on bodily sensations. Running on the treadmill was the slowest, but felt hardest, most likely because the unstimulating environment meant there was little else to pay attention to other than how they were feeling, amplifying these sensations and increasing how hard the run felt as a result. In contrast, running the more stimulating outdoor route was not only faster, but felt the easiest. This finding, that our attention can impact how we feel, has further implications that we'll explore later in this chapter.

FOCUSING ON RUNNING TECHNIQUE

Focusing on our running technique can also improve running performance and help us deal with sensations of effort. When running faster is our aim, focusing on elements of our running technique, such as our stride or arm drive, is more effective than distraction. We can help to direct our focus using instructional self-talk statements like those we introduced in Chapter 3. To highlight the benefits of this approach, two studies led by psychologist Brad Donohue provide an insight into the effects of a running-technique focus on performance.

In the first study, Donohue and colleagues (Donohue et al., 2001) found that a group of six female cross-country runners who used instructional cues to help them focus on actions that would likely result in an optimum performance (such as, "get an explosive start," "strike heels against ground softly," or "run through the finish line") had the greatest improvement in 1,000m times (improved by 19 seconds relative to baseline) in comparison to when they repeated motivational statements only such as, "You're going to dominate today" or "You've worked hard for this" (improved by 17 seconds), and when focused on their naturally occurring thoughts and feelings (improved by 12 seconds).

In a follow-up study, 30 high school middle-distance runners who received a combination of personalised, instructional/running technique statements (for example, "Keep your eyes focused ahead"; "Keep hands open and relaxed") and motivational statements (for example, "This is what you've been training for"; "Let's go, let's do it") significantly improved their one-mile running performance by eight seconds in comparison with a pre-intervention run. A separate group of 30 runners that listened to motivational music while they ran also significantly improved their performance, in this instance by five seconds. But a final group of 30 runners who received no intervention only improved by two seconds—a non-significant change from baseline (Miller & Donohue, 2003).

These findings add to what we learned about motivational self-talk in Chapter 3. More so, these studies highlight that statements which provide instructions to focus on pacing, and on running form or technique, can help us run faster. Using both motivational and instructional self-talk in combination can be an effective strategy to optimise running performance when needed.

ATTENTION AND RUNNING ECONOMY

Although tuning in periodically and using cues to optimise our running technique can improve performance, some studies have highlighted that what we focus on can also impact on our running economy. As we learned in Chapter 3, running economy is a measure of how efficient a runner is based on the amount of oxygen their body uses when running at a specific pace. Alongside our VO_{2max} and lactate threshold, running economy is an important physiological variable that determines running performance.

Many psychological factors can influence our running economy. In one study, changes in mood, and specifically higher tension, depression, anger, or confusion, and lower feelings of energy/vigour, were associated with worse running economy (Williams et al., 1991). But what we focus our attention on can also impact on how efficiently we run. In a series of studies, University of Münster researcher Linda Schücker has shown that when we focus on highly automated processes, such as our running movement or our breathing, we tend to be *less* efficient as a consequence. In one study, asking runners to focus their attention on either their breathing mechanics or on their running movement (by instructing them to "focus on the forward movement of your legs") resulted in less-efficient running and a higher heart rate than focusing on feelings of effort or on their normal thoughts (Schücker et al., 2014).

Other studies with a similar design have shown that focusing either on the mechanics of breathing or on leg movements result in poorer running economy than focusing on one's usual running thoughts, or focusing attention externally, such as on the surroundings (Hill et al., 2017). One psychological theory to explain why focusing attention on monitoring our movements or our breathing is detrimental is the *constrained-action hypothesis* (Wulf et al., 2001). This theory suggests that when we consciously focus internally on monitoring movements or processes that occur automatically, like our leg action or our breathing, automatic control is disrupted, and our movements become less efficient as a result. Focusing on feelings of effort does not have the same impact since our sense of "effort" is not an automatic process. As such, for most runners, tuning out from monitoring running movements and letting them happen naturally might be best for more-efficient running.

The findings of these studies seem to contradict those of Brad Donohue and colleagues who found that using cues related to running technique led to improvements in running performance. One subtle difference, however, relates to what runners focused on. In the studies performed by Schücker and colleagues, runners simply monitored "the forward movement of their legs"—something that we don't tend to focus on in reality. In the Donohue studies, however, runners focused on optimising their technique and running form. In this way, the advice to focus on "keeping your hands open and relaxed" or "pumping your arms" is much more likely to optimise movement technique and help running performance than simply monitoring the forward movement of your legs.

MINDFULNESS AND RUNNING PERFORMANCE

As an attentional strategy, mindfulness involves paying attention, on purpose, in the present moment. Much like association, being mindful means having an awareness of our internal experiences, such as our thoughts or feelings, and external stimuli, such as objects in our surrounding environment. As a psychological technique, however, mindfulness does not involve changing our thoughts or experiences in the same way that a motivational self-talk intervention or reappraisal does. Instead, being mindful means that we accept experiences, such as negative thoughts or sensations of effort, in a non-judgemental way.

There are many mindfulness protocols, but one that has received some attention with runners is the Mindful Sport Performance Enhancement programme (MSPE; Kaufman et al., 2009). The MSPE protocol was originally developed for golfers and archers, and involves between four and six sessions with activities including mindful breathing exercises, body scanning, and sport-specific mindfulness exercises adapted for any sport. For runners, the purpose of these activities is to develop skills to deal with running-specific challenges, such as staying focused in the present moment, overcoming distractions, accepting sensations of effort or pain as a natural part of the running experience, and letting negative thoughts pass without judgement. The sport-specific aspects of MSPE training can help runners prepare for individual points of a race, such as reaching a mile marker or completing the race, with a reminder to stay focused or to maintain running form at each point.

Research on the impact of mindfulness training with runners shows some positive effects, but this evidence is based on some low-quality studies (Corbally et al., 2020). Mindfulness training has been shown to improve scores on measures of state mindfulness, for example. One study demonstrated that runners who completed MSPE training improved their ability to "defuse"—a mental skill that includes accepting and separating ourselves from our thoughts and feelings. Mindfulness training has also been shown to reduce sport-specific feelings of anxiety, perfectionism, and worry with runners (Hut et al., 2021).

In terms of performance, no studies have shown that mindfulness training helps runners go faster. No differences in running performance as measured by best mile times were shown after MSPE training in one study (De Petrillo et al., 2009). A longer-term follow-up of that study did note that runners were faster one year after receiving the mindfulness training, but whether the improvement was due to the mindfulness intervention or training over the course of the year could not be determined (Thompson et al., 2011). Finally, in comparison with baseline measures, a group of female college runners who underwent eight weeks of mindfulness training demonstrated improvements in measures of psychological resilience and reported lower perceptions of effort following an 800m run (Wang et al., 2021). However, that study failed to report the 800m performance times of runners, casting doubt on whether the lower perceived effort coincided with equal or faster running times.

While mindful practice is intuitively appealing as a technique to help runners focus their attention during training or racing, there is a lack of good-quality research on mindfulness training with runners. The general conclusion is that mindfulness training may improve state mindfulness and might also reduce feelings of anxiety and worry, both helpful changes for runners. But whether this translates to faster running performance is unclear.

DISTRACTION: TUNING OUT TO FEEL GOOD

Similar to an associative-type focus, distraction can be both helpful and unhelpful for runners. In terms of benefits, distraction can help runners tune out from unpleasant sensations or feelings, especially at lower running intensities. At any one time, the amount of information we can pay attention to, and process, is limited. Because of this, being distracted by our own thoughts or by scenic views, for example, can reduce our awareness of unpleasant bodily sensations. As a result, running can feel easier and more pleasant. Distraction can be especially useful when running quickly isn't the primary goal. The distraction that results from running in nature settings, for example, like a green park or along a beach, can increase enjoyment and reduce feelings of boredom. Focusing on scenic views can also improve our mood, helping to lower tension and increase feelings of vigour after a run (Butryn & Furst, 2003).

Distraction can also help runners experience flow, an optimal, enjoyable experience where we become totally immersed in a task and our attention and focus feel effortless. We (Jackman et al., 2021) found that when an outdoor training run involved variety or novelty, such as exploring a new running route or when the main objective was to enjoy the run, runners were more likely to experience flow. More so, what these runners focused their attention on was different during flow states. Typically, runners did not monitor their watch or device, and did not use any strategies like motivational self-talk, chunking, or focus on their running technique. Instead, they distracted themselves by focusing on the surrounding views, listening to music, engaging in conversations with others, or generally switching-off and letting their mind wander as they ran. As a result, these runners reported feeling better and enjoying their run more and described it as an experience that they didn't want to end.

These positive benefits aside, distraction can also be unhelpful for runners. Distraction, as the early work of Morgan and Pollock hinted at, is something that runners try to avoid when attempting to perform at their best. When we are distracted, whether intentionally or involuntarily, our pace is typically slower than it is when we are focused on running-related thoughts and actions. For competitive runners, this can have an immediate impact on their performance. One international-level cross-country runner that we interviewed (Brick et al., 2015) gave this example to highlight the detrimental impact of distraction on race performance:

> I went through 2 [kilometers] and 4 [kilometers] on the back of the leading group. And going into the third lap, I started falling off the leading group. And it was everything for me to stay attached [because I was distracted by a spectator] and suddenly I just lost a second's concentration, and it was like, 'Don't lose concentration, concentrate now,' and I covered the move. I finished second in that race. But if I had fallen off that group, I wouldn't have gotten back on and that would have been it.

What these findings show is that when running fast is a priority, distraction should be avoided in favour of a focus on task-relevant thoughts and actions. When our primary aim is to feel good and enjoy the experience of running, however, distraction can be especially useful. In addition to focusing on our surroundings, one way that many runners choose to distract themselves is by listening to music. But music can have many different benefits for runners, not just helping to provide a distraction, but also helping to improve running performance. In the next section, we will explore the impact of listening to music on our running activity.

CAN MUSIC HELP MY RUNNING ACTIVITY?

In sport and exercise broadly, music can have multiple benefits. Music can increase affective valence, meaning that we feel better when listening to music during exercise. Music has also been shown to enhance performance, help make activities feel easier, and improve movement efficiency (Terry et al., 2020). When using music during running, four musical factors are important. Foremost amongst these are the musical qualities of *rhythm* (such as the tempo of the song in beats per minute), *harmony*, and *melody*. Also important are the *cultural impact* and the *associations* we have with a piece of music, including the memories or emotions that the music evokes. Each of these factors determine the motivational qualities of a piece of music and how it might impact on our running performance (Terry & Karageorghis, 2006).

Most research with runners has focused on the effects of *asynchronous music*, that is, music to which our footsteps are not coordinated. Based on extensive research and reviews led by University of Brunel psychologist Costas Karageorghis, we have learned that listening to asynchronous music when running leads to higher enjoyment, more pleasant feelings, and lower perceptions of effort in comparison to running without music (Karageorghis & Priest, 2012a). This is particularly true for less-experienced runners and when running at moderate or low intensities. When listening to music at a self-selected "feel good" pace, for example, people tend to run faster and, despite this faster pace, report running as feeling more pleasant with music than without (Hutchinson et al., 2018). When used to help make running feel easier or more pleasant, the ideal tempo for asynchronous music seems to fall between 120–140bpm, regardless of intensity. Think of Ed Sheeran's "Bad Habits" at 126bpm or Darude's "Sandstorm" at 138bpm as examples of songs within this range. However, our musical preferences are also important, and preferred music is better than non-preferred music to help make running feel easier and more pleasant (Ballmann, 2021).

Interestingly, music can also play an important role during easy or recovery runs. Listening to classical music, for example, has been shown to lower heart rate and blood pressure when running (Szmedra & Bacharach, 1998) and relaxing, sedative music can play a similar role to help recovery as part of a post-run cooldown. Findings on the effects of music at higher intensity, hard-pace running is less consistent. In one study, when running at 90% of VO_{2max}, a pace that most runners could sustain for about 12 minutes before stopping, neither rock, dance, nor inspirational (such as Survivor's "Eye of the

Tiger") music helped to make running feel easier or improve performance (Tenenbaum et al., 2004). Similar findings were noted in the same study when participants completed a series of 2.2km runs as fast as possible; music did not help to improve performance or lower perceptions of effort. As highlighted earlier in this chapter, one reason that music may be less effective at higher intensities is that bodily sensations dominate our focus of attention, and it is harder for music to distract us from these physiological cues (Tenenbaum, 2001).

Despite this, other factors, such as the motivational qualities of a piece of music and our dominant attentional style, might be more important when it comes to higher-intensity running. In terms of attentional style, some studies have suggested that we can be grouped into one of three categories based on a scale called the Attentional Focus Questionnaire (Brewer et al., 1996). Based on Morgan and Pollock's early work on attentional focus, if, during a maximal effort endurance run, you are inclined to pay attention to your general level of fatigue, focus on staying loose and relaxed, or encourage yourself to run fast, then you are an "associator." If you are more likely sing a song in your head, focus on the scenery, or try to ignore physical sensations, then you are a "dissociator." If it is somewhere in-between, then you are a "switcher." Psychologists Jasmine Hutchinson and Costas Karageorghis noted that, when listening to motivational music or non-motivational music versus no music, all individuals in their study were distracted by music when running at a low intensity. At moderate intensity, however, runners tended to adopt their dominant style; the dissociators were more distracted by non-motivational music, whereas the associators focused more on how they felt or on staying loose, and so forth. Finally, at the highest intensity of running, all groups became more associative when listening to motivational music (Hutchinson & Karageorghis, 2013).

What this study shows is that intensity, and our preferred attentional style, are both important to determine the effects of music on running performance. Music helped runners distract themselves at lower intensities, and this can be helpful to reduce boredom and make running feel more enjoyable during slower-paced runs. While runners adopted their preferred focus at moderate intensities, motivational music helped all runners focus more on their movements, staying relaxed, and so on at the highest intensity. As a result, the researchers suggested that motivational music has the potential to help us perform better during high-intensity running. This means carefully selecting music that you find motivating if running at a harder pace. To do so, choose music with a rhythm, style, melody, tempo, sound, beat, or lyrics that you find personally motivating.

Studies have also explored the effects of *synchronous music*, that is, music to which we consciously coordinate our footsteps in time with the beat when running (Karageorghis & Priest, 2012b). In 400m running time-trials, synchronous music led to faster times relative to a no-music run, regardless of whether that music was considered motivational or not (Simpson & Karageorghis, 2006). Similarly, elite triathletes have been shown to last 78 seconds (18.1%) longer when listening to synchronous, motivational music, and 85 seconds longer (19.7%) when listening to synchronous, neutral (non-motivating) music during a run-to-exhaustion trial (Terry et al., 2012). In line with findings for asynchronous music, perceived effort was also lower when listening to music versus no-music, regardless of its motivational properties. Similar findings have also been shown when running in hot (31°C) and humid (70%) conditions, with runners lasting 66.59% longer (approx. 2.5 minutes) when running at 80% of their VO_{2max} listening to synchronous music versus no music (Nikol et al., 2018).

Interestingly, in line with findings from other activities, runners in the Terry et al. (2012) study were also more efficient when synchronising their movements to the music and used less oxygen as a result, suggesting that synchronous music can also help to improve running economy. It may be that running movements become more rhythmic when coordinated with a piece of carefully selected music. Collectively, these studies show that synchronising our movements to a piece of music can improve performance, make running feel easier, and improve the efficiency of our running movements.

KEY POINTS ON ATTENTION DURING RUNNING

1. A runners' attentional focus is variable, flexible, and dynamic. Runners focus on lots of different things, and each of these impacts running performance and how we feel.

2. Focusing excessively on bodily sensations can make running feel harder. Instead, tune in periodically. Perform a body scan (for example, how's my breathing, how do my shoulders feel) and use this as a source of information to adjust your running pace, to relax your upper body, and so forth.

3. Faster performance results from using association-type strategies. Use strategies like relaxation or instructional cues to focus on optimising running technique and to run faster.

4. Monitoring automatic processes, like breathing mechanics and running movements, can result in less-efficient running, especially for experienced runners. Avoid monitoring these processes excessively.

5. Avoid distraction if your goal is to run fast. But distraction can help make running feel easier, more pleasant, and more enjoyable. Helpful distractions include chatting with a running partner, focusing on scenic nature views, or letting your mind wander.

6. If using music, choose music based on what you want from a run (for example, distraction, relaxation, or motivation) and choose music that you prefer. Asynchronous music helps improve running performance and can make running feel easier, more pleasant, and more enjoyable. Synchronous music can also help improve running economy.

7. For motivation, choose music with a rhythm, style, melody, tempo, sound, beat, or lyrics that you find personally motivating.

8. If using music, stay safe and avoid using music if running on a road!

RUN WITH IT: HOW CAN I MAKE RUNNING FEEL MORE PLEASANT?

When we first started to work with Angela, she was struggling to stay motivated to complete her weekly running sessions. Angela took up running aged 45, following a recommendation by her doctor to increase her physical activity levels. She began running on a local Couch to 5k programme but, two months after finishing the programme, felt that she was still overweight, could not run very fast, and hated how loud her breathing sounded when she ran. As this point, she began to dislike running and wanted to quit. However, she also wanted to continue her running journey. She recognised the health benefits that it brought, and she had noticed some improvements in her speed and times from when she first started on the Couch to 5k programme. She also appreciated the time alone during running to distract herself from a stressful job and a busy family life. But, despite these benefits, she just wasn't enjoying running as much as she had when she started.

In our first chat with Angela, we started to work through why she wanted to stop. A few key points emerged. First, toward the end of the Couch to 5k programme, she had become more focused on running faster times and being competitive. She would often compare herself to other runners and feel like she had to try to beat them. She also paid more attention to her pace and became obsessed with looking at her watch during a run. If she was behind others, or ran slower than she thought she should, it often left her feeling frustrated and deflated after a training session or a 5k parkrun. She also hated the sound of her breathing and felt very self-conscious when running with others because of how she felt she sounded. What became clear from this first session was that Angela's motives for running had shifted toward more extrinsic, controlled forms of motivation (see Chapter 1). Her goals were more performance (time) and outcome-based (beating others), and she spent a lot of time tuning in to bodily sensations, like her breathing. Each of these were beginning to make running an unpleasant experience for Angela.

We worked with Angela to incorporate several new psychological strategies into her training. First, we began by exploring why running was important to Angela and why she wanted to continue running for the long-term. On the top of her list was that she wanted to be fit and healthy, that running helped her to de-stress and lift her mood, and she also wanted to set a good example for her children. This helped Angela notice that her main reasons for running were very different to the more extrinsic reasons that she now focused on, and that these were beginning to undermine her enjoyment of her running sessions.

To help shift Angela away from a focus on running at a set pace or trying to beat others, we encouraged Angela to focus on more "open" goals in training. This might be to run as fast as she wanted to, or to run for as long as she wanted to in training runs. We also encouraged Angela to run some sessions without a watch and without the pressure of focusing on her pace or distance. Ultimately, she decided to leave her watch behind on some sessions only, as she also liked to see some improvements, like running a new furthest distance. But on these "watch-less" sessions, her focus was to enjoy simply being able to run.

We also explored where Angela liked to run. Living in the countryside, she found running in this area more pleasant and enjoyable, and it helped to take her mind off how she was feeling and, specifically, her breathing sensations. She also felt that running in the countryside helped her to destress from her busy lifestyle. We encouraged Angela to explore safe running routes around her home in the countryside and to explore new routes when possible. But she wasn't always able to run in these settings. Sometimes it was too dark, or felt unsafe, and, on these occasions, she ran on an indoor treadmill at home. These were some of her least favourite sessions, where there was "nothing to focus on but four grey walls and the sound of my breathing over the treadmill!" For these treadmill runs, we worked with Angela to develop a music playlist that she would enjoy and that would help her running experience. We selected music that she liked, that included some lyrics that she found motivational, and, for some songs, had a tempo suitable for running. Songs from her playlist included Florence and the Machine's "Dog Days are Over", U2's "Where the Streets Have No Name," and David Guetta's "Titanium" ft. Sia. We recommended that Angela run at a "feel good" pace when listening to these songs on the treadmill, and to ignore the pace display on the treadmill.

For each run, whether in the countryside alone, at her local parkrun, or on the treadmill with music playing, we asked Angela to keep a diary and to take note of two or three things that she noticed during the run and a further two or three good things that she noticed after the run. Below are examples from one countryside run and one treadmill run. These helped Angela remind herself of what she enjoyed about running, what felt good about running, and the benefits she perceived she got from running. This strategy also helped to shift her focus away from some aspects that had undermined this enjoyment, such as being competitive or overly focused on times.

Table 4.1 Entries from Angela's running diary following one countryside run and one treadmill run.

	2km run alone near home	2 X 1.5km runs on treadmill
During the run	So peaceful and quiet. Took my mind off work.	Didn't want to run, so set out to start and "see what I could do."
	Was getting dark near the end, but the stars were coming out. Saw the moon rising—amazing!	Loved the tunes. Got me into a bouncy rhythm. "I want to run."
	Slow, but didn't care.	Wanted to do a third run, but didn't have the time.
After the run	Felt much more relaxed in the evening.	Felt energised by the music.
	Slept well that night.	In a good mood with family!

Angela enjoyed setting open goals for some of her runs and felt that this focus took away some of the pressure that she was putting on herself to run faster or to beat other people. She also enjoyed not wearing her watch sometimes, especially on the countryside runs around home where she preferred just to get out, enjoy the views around her, have some time to herself, and not worry about her time or pace. Because of this, she felt she often "switched off" during these runs and went further than she otherwise would. She began to wear a watch again on some of these runs to track her distance because "I wanted to see how far I ran, not because I felt I had to run a certain distance or pace, but because I was curious. I didn't look at my pace during those runs." She also felt that music helped make the treadmill runs more enjoyable, as there was something else to focus on. More so, it also helped her to tune out from her breathing.

Since this time, Angela has maintained her running and, though predominantly running for fitness and enjoyment, has started to enter more races. She would classify herself as a "back of the pack" runner and, although she likes to note her times, her focus now is to enjoy her running experiences. That might include chatting with others or offering encouragement, running faster if she feels she wants to, or taking in the views, especially in some off-road trail races she did in the past few months. As she has gotten fitter, her breathing has also improved and doesn't distract her like it once did. After one recent race, Angela reflected that:

> I can be running along merrily and I remember how hard I found my first few runs or how I was beginning to lose my love for running by focusing on the wrong things for me. I am truly amazed at how far I have come.

5

CAN RUNNING HELP ME FEEL BETTER?

INTRODUCTION

When compared with non-runners, runners report better mental health and higher psychological wellbeing. Runners tend to score lower on measures of anxiety and depression, for example, and report better mood. But how much running do we need to do to gain these benefits, and do these benefits persist over time? In this chapter we will provide an overview of the mental health benefits of running and provide practical suggestions on how much running you need to do in terms of frequency, intensity, and duration to gain these benefits.

Running also challenges our brain in many ways. As we introduced in Chapter 1, the cognitive challenges imposed by running mean that our brain adapts and many brain functions, like memory and attention, improve as a result of running. These findings suggest that running can improve brain health across the lifespan, reduce or reverse age-related decline in brain function, and lower our risk of dementia. In this chapter, we will also delve deeper into this research and explore the effects of aerobic exercise, like running, on the health of our brain.

Finally, despite these many benefits, there is also a darker side to running. Although running can be an enjoyable activity that many people dedicate a large amount of time to participate in, for others,

DOI: 10.4324/9781003204206-6

running can control their lives, often to the detriment of social relationships and work responsibilities. Toward the end of this chapter, we will explore exercise addiction, outline how you might assess your risk of exercise addiction, and clarify what you can do if you are concerned about your running behaviours.

We will begin this chapter with some insights on the impact of running on mental health and provide answers to a seemingly straightforward question: "Can running help me feel better?" First, we will explain what we mean by the mental health outcomes associated with running.

WHAT ARE MENTAL HEALTH OUTCOMES?

Mental health outcomes relevant for running include anxiety, depression, our mood state, and psychological wellbeing. In the table that follows, we have provided a brief description of a range of mental health outcomes to fully explain some of the measures of mental health that we will explore in this chapter.

In the following sections, we will delve into the impact of running under two broad areas: 1) the effects of a single bout of running on mental health outcomes; and 2) the effects of longer term running, such as weeks or months of activity, on mental health outcomes.

CAN A SINGLE BOUT OF RUNNING CHANGE HOW I FEEL?

To explore the effects of running on how we feel, researchers typically compare people's mental health, mood, or psychological wellbeing before and after a single session of running. The broad finding is that a single session of running can have a positive effect on how we feel. Thirty to 40 minutes of running has been shown to reduce feelings of anxiety and depression, improve mood, and increase psychological wellbeing in comparison with pre-run states, for example. In one study, 30 minutes of vigorous intensity running—a pace at between 70% to 90% of your maximum heart rate that will feel

Table 5.1 Description of key mental health outcomes included in this chapter (adapted from Oswald et al., 2020).

Outcome	Description
Anxiety	Anxiety is characterised by uncomfortable or upsetting thoughts and is usually accompanied by feelings of agitation and tension. Anxiety includes transient anxiety symptoms (called state anxiety), more persistent symptoms (called trait anxiety), and clinical disorders characterised by excessive, chronic anxiety. Examples of anxiety disorders are social phobia, generalised anxiety disorder, panic disorder, obsessive-compulsive disorder, and post-traumatic stress disorder.
Depression	Depression is a mood disorder with prolonged periods of low mood and a lack of interest and/or pleasure in normal activities most of the time. This includes major depressive disorder.
Mood	Mood is a transient state of a set of feelings that can vary in intensity and duration. In the studies reported in this chapter, the moods most often measured are tension/anxiety, depression, anger, fatigue, and confusion as negative mood states and feelings of vigour/energy as a positive mood state. Total Mood Disturbance is the sum score of these negative moods minus feelings of vigour, with higher scores indicating a worse mood.
Psychological stress/ distress	Psychological stress or distress is a discomforting emotional state experienced in response to a specific stressor or demand that results in harm, either temporary or permanent, to a person.
Psychological wellbeing	Psychological wellbeing links with a sense of choice/autonomy, mastery (for example, of a running task), personal growth, positive relationships with others, purpose in life, and self-acceptance. This is also referred to as eudemonic wellbeing.
Self-esteem	Self-esteem is the feeling of value and worth that a person has for themselves. Self-esteem contributes to overall self-concept, or the qualities that we attribute to ourselves (for example, what we see as our strengths and qualities).

somewhat hard—led to higher feelings of energy, lower state anxiety, lower feelings of depression, fatigue, and confusion, and improved mood post-run (McDowell et al., 2016). Interestingly, the magnitude of changes in anxiety and mood states post-run were greater amongst women than men for most of these outcomes. One reason for this was that the women in this study reported a worse mood pre-run than men did, suggesting that running can have a bigger positive impact on how we feel for those who feel worse to begin with.

Several factors impact how a single bout of running changes how we feel. The first factor is how long we need to run to gain some benefits. Most studies have asked people to run for between 30 minutes and 60 minutes, or to run distances between 5km and 10km, and these studies generally report positive effects on mood, symptoms of anxiety and depression, and psychological wellbeing. But running for even shorter durations can have positive effects. In one study, ten minutes of light-intensity jogging outdoors improved the mood of regular exercisers when compared with spending the same period of time at rest (Anderson & Brice, 2011). In another study, 20 minutes of track running at a self-selected pace helped to reduce feelings of anxiety in university students (Szabo, 2003). Finally, 25 minutes of vigorous intensity running led to improvements in depressed mood immediately afterwards in people with a clinical diagnosis of depressive disorder in comparison with people with no such diagnosis. These changes were short-lived, however, and 30 minutes after finishing their run, participants reported higher levels of depression and fatigue and lower feelings of energy/vigour (Weinstein et al., 2010). What these studies and others tell us is that even a short bout of running, as little as ten to 20 minutes, helps to improve how we feel, but these changes can be short-lived and gradually return to pre-run levels soon after we finish a run.

A second factor that impacts on how we feel after running is the intensity or pace at which we run. In one study, walking or running for 20 minutes at moderate or vigorous intensities, ranging from 55% to 79% of maximum heart rate, led to improvements in mood post-run (Berger & Owen, 1998). However, higher intensity running, that is running at a pace that feels hard or very hard, can lead us to feel more, rather than less, anxious immediately afterwards. In another study, 20 minutes of walking or running at both 5% below the lactate threshold and at the lactate threshold intensity led to lower feelings of anxiety that lasted up to one-hour post-run. However, when participants ran for 20 minutes at a higher intensity, 5% above their lactate threshold, feelings of anxiety *increased* in the 30-minute period post-run before eventually decreasing to below pre-run levels 45 minutes post-run (Markowitz & Arent, 2010). (See the *Affective States* Section in Chapter 2 as a reminder of why the lactate threshold is an important intensity landmark.) These findings suggest that higher-intensity running requires a longer period, about 30 minutes, to recover from and, during this recovery period, higher body temperature, an elevated heart rate, and a faster breathing rate—all symptoms of anxiety— can mean that we perceive higher anxiety levels immediately after a higher-intensity run. Lower-intensity running, such as running at a pace that feels light or somewhat hard and that allows you to speak comfortably or complete short sentences before needing to take a breath, does not seem to have the same impact and can lead to lower feelings of anxiety post-run instead.

One final factor that impacts how we feel post-run is *where* we choose to run. This might be in a nature setting, such as a trail or park, in an urban setting such as an industrial or shopping area, or indoors on a treadmill. Although running in both nature and urban settings can lead to positive changes in mood, runners often prefer nature settings and report greater feelings of calmness, relaxation, and psychological restoration (that is, feeling like they had a mental break from day-to-day routines) after running in nature in comparison with urban settings (Butryn & Furst, 2003). Running indoors on a treadmill versus outdoors can also lead to similar effects. Specifically, moderate-intensity running that feels light or somewhat hard, whether on a treadmill or outdoors, can lead to increases in pleasant feelings, such as feeling relaxed or excited, and decreases in unpleasant feelings, such as feeling anxiety and anger (Kerr et al., 2006). However, running outdoors has also been shown to lead to greater improvements in mood such as lower anxiety, depression, anger, and fatigue, and higher energy than after a treadmill run (Harte & Eifert, 1995; LaCaille et al., 2004). Overall, what these studies show is that running, regardless of location, can improve how we feel. But running outdoors in nature settings can be more satisfying and lead to even greater improvements in how we feel than running in urban settings or running indoors on a treadmill.

The benefits of running for how we feel broadly aligns with those on the effects of other types of exercise (Reed & Ones, 2006). That is, the effects are mostly positive immediately after exercise and are greatest for those who feel worse beforehand. The positive effects generally last for at least 30 minutes after exercise before gradually returning to pre-exercise levels. But exercise intensity and duration—together known as *exercise dose*—also play a role. The ideal for runners to maximise how good you feel afterwards appears to be no more than 40 minutes at a comfortable pace below 70% of your maximum heart rate (this pace feels light or somewhat hard, and you should be able to speak comfortably throughout). If you prefer to go a little faster, then run for no more than 20–30 minutes at a pace below 90% of your maximum heart rate (this pace feels somewhat hard to hard, and you can only speak short or broken sentences). High exercise doses, such as 60–90 minutes of moderate intensity or 40–60 minutes of high-intensity activity, are still beneficial but have less of a positive effect on how we feel. Very high doses, such as very long runs or running at a hard to very hard pace can have a negative effect on how we feel afterwards. Running outdoors in a nature setting can add to the positive effects of running on how we feel.

To find your own sweet spot, you can explore the effects of running on your mood using valid assessment tools. One measure is called the Brunel Mood Scale (Terry et al., 2003) and an online version can be found at www.moodprofiling.com/. Take a few minutes to complete the mood scale before a run and take note of your results. Complete the scale once again after you run. Did you notice any changes in your mood after running versus before? Were these changes positive or negative? How long did these changes last after you finished the run? Using the same mood scale, you can compare runs of different durations (for example, ten minutes versus 30 minutes), intensities (for example, easy, light pace versus hard or very hard pace), and locations (for example, treadmill versus an outdoor park or trail setting) to build a clearer picture of how running impacts how you feel.

CAN LONGER-TERM RUNNING CHANGE HOW I FEEL?

Longer-term running, that is, consistent running over weeks and months, can provide further benefits for how we feel. Those who run regularly generally report more positive moods, lower anxiety, and lower depression on running days than on non-running days. But taking up running for the first time can also provide a boost. One study compared the effects of a three-week running programme on mood (both on waking and at bedtime), perceived stress, sleep quality, and concentration in a group of adolescents (Kalak et al., 2012). Half of the group completed a 30-minute self-paced morning run every weekday before school started, whereas the remaining "non-runners" spent this time at rest, chatting to other study participants or doing homework. At the end of the three-week period, those in the running group had higher sleep quality, felt in a better mood in the morning when they woke, and reported improved concentration and lower sleepiness over the three-week programme. This highlights that as little as three weeks of running can lead to noticeable improvements in many aspects of how we feel.

Longer-term running can also lead to more persistent effects. In studies that used walking/running programmes lasting anywhere between eight and 20 weeks in duration, and that typically consisted of at least two or three 20–30-minute runs per week, significant improvements were shown for mood and self-esteem, lower symptoms of anxiety and depression, and an improved ability to deal with stressful life events (Von Haaren et al., 2015). Similar to findings for single bouts of running, running at a moderate intensity and comfortable pace leads to greater improvements in longer-term mental health than higher-intensity running, especially for beginners (Moses et al., 1989). One reason for this may be that moderate-intensity running is more manageable and enjoyable for beginners and leads to better mental health outcomes as a result. For regular runners, however, such as those training for a half-marathon or a full marathon, a different pattern seems to exist. For these more experienced runners with a goal to aim for, running more often each week (such as on six or seven days) can lead to better psychological wellbeing and greater feelings of satisfaction with life. Running further distances in training can also increase self-esteem and lead to a greater sense of meaning in life, possibly due to feelings of accomplishment gained from running longer distances and achieving training or race-related goals (Nezlek et al., 2018).

Running, like other forms of exercise, such as walking or resistance training, is also beneficial for those with a mental health condition like anxiety or depression (Schuch et al., 2016; Shannon et al., 2023). Eight weeks of moderate intensity walking/running training in a nature setting, completed for 30–45 minutes on three days per week, led to lower symptoms of depression in male and female participants with a pre-existing diagnosis of mild or moderate depression, for example (Doose et al., 2015). But that's not to say that running works for everyone. Maintaining the motivation to complete a longer-term running programme can be challenging, including for those with mental health conditions, with one study reporting that 81% of individuals with major depressive disorder dropped out of a twice-weekly walking/running programme by the end of a six-month period (Kruisdijk et al., 2012).

Based on the existing evidence base, the advice for long-term running is that any running, or exercise in general, can improve how we feel (Reed & Buck, 2009). For each session, follow the guidelines from the previous section on the intensity and duration of each run. During each week, run as often as you wish. Some running is better than none, but three or more sessions per week may lead to greater improvements in how you feel than fewer sessions. Most well-designed programmes follow a progressive training plan that increases running frequency, intensity, or duration as your fitness improves. Following a recognised training plan, such as a Couch to 5k programme, will help if you are a beginner runner. You can search online for a Couch to 5k running plan or download the Couch to 5k app on your mobile device. Your local running club might also offer a Couch to 5k or similar programme for beginners.

It may take some time to notice longer-term improvements in your mood, psychological wellbeing, or symptoms of anxiety and depression, but changes can be evident within as little as a few weeks of consistent running a few times per week. You can run indoors or outdoors, and by yourself or with others. If you do run with a group, your relationship with other group members can provide some additional benefits to your mental health. Higher levels of friendship with other members of a running group can lead to lower anxiety, depression, and stress (Keating et al., 2018). Running buddies can also help us stick with running longer-term. As such, doing some of your weekly runs with friends can help to further improve how you feel and keep you on track with your running activity. In Chapter 6, we will explore these social benefits further when we focus on programmes with a running element such as Girls on the Run and parkrun.

WHY DOES RUNNING HELP US FEEL BETTER?

There are several biological and psychological reasons to explain the effects of running on how we feel. From a biological perspective, running changes the levels of multiple chemicals in our brain known as *neurotransmitters*. Neurotransmitters are chemical messengers, and their job is to carry signals from one nerve cell to another. In doing so, they regulate how our body, and our brain, functions. We know of over 100 neurotransmitters, and each plays a different role such as to activate us or calm us down, to regulate our sleep-wake cycle, to help us concentrate and focus, or to amplify or dull our experience of pain. Neurotransmitters also change how we feel and help regulate our emotions, our motivation, and our mood. Importantly, physical activities like running also impact on the neurotransmitters released by our nerve cells and, by doing so, change how we feel. Running can cause changes in levels of a range of neurotransmitters, but the two that have received most attention are serotonin and dopamine. Serotonin increases after exercise—especially low- or moderate-intensity activity—and changes in serotonin levels are linked with the anxiety-reducing and anti-depression effects of exercise. Similarly, levels of dopamine can also increase after a single bout of activity and dopamine is linked with feelings of motivation for exercise and the rewarding, feel-good effects we experience after exercise (Basso & Suzuki, 2017).

Running also impacts a range of chemicals called *neuromodulators*. These chemicals impact the amount of a neurotransmitter that is produced by a nerve cell and, by doing so, are part of a chain of events that can change how we feel. Perhaps one of the most widely known theories of how running boosts our mood is called the *endorphin hypothesis*. Endorphins—naturally occurring chemicals in our body that can help to relieve pain—are often promoted as the cause of the *runner's high*, a feeling of elation, peacefulness, boundless energy, and lower pain sensation that we might experience after a run. Whether the runner's high exists or not is open to question, however, with some runners reporting an experience of it, others not, and some experiencing it only rarely. But running does help us feel better, and one reason for this is that we experience a natural "reward" after running that motivates more running behaviour for a longer term. Given the importance of running in our evolutionary history (see Chapter 1), and the effort and energy cost associated with running, having some natural means to motivate us to run more is clearly important. Whether endorphins play a role in this feel-good sensation after running is contentious, however, with findings that endorphins circulating in our bloodstream after running—a key measure taken by researchers—are too big to cross a barrier that controls what chemicals can enter our brain. As a result, the commonly held belief that endorphins underpin the runner's high is problematic because endorphins found in our bloodstream after running may have little impact on the chemistry of our brain and on how we feel after running (Dietrich & McDaniel, 2004).

More recent attention has shifted to a second group of neuromodulators called *endocannabinoids* (Sparling et al., 2003). Endocannabinoids are produced naturally by our body and have a similar effect as cannabis, leading to a more sedate, relaxed state and higher feelings of wellbeing. These chemicals can also cross the barrier from our blood-stream into our brain and are capable of changing activity in our brain as a result. Endocannabinoids are produced when we run, and higher levels of endocannabinoids lead to the release of dopamine in areas of our brain that ultimately results in some of the pleasant and rewarding feelings associated with running. Endocannabinoids also lower pain sensitivity, helping runners to tolerate exercise-induced pain during activity. Interestingly, endocannabinoids are produced during running in both humans and in running dogs, but not in animals that don't run very much like ferrets, suggesting that the production of endocannabinoids, and the "rewarding" feelings experienced as a result, is specific to species like humans and dogs that specialised in long-distance running during their evolution (Raichlen et al., 2012). The production of endocannabinoids is also dependent on the intensity of activity, and endocannabinoid levels increase after moderate- and vigorous-intensity running, but not after very-high-intensity running (>90% of maximum heart rate) or very-low-intensity activity, like walking. These findings match those suggesting that moderate-intensity running leads to the greatest improvements in how we feel after activity (Raichlen et al., 2013). Taken together, these studies provide compelling evidence for the role that endocannabinoids might play to improve how we feel after running. One type of endocannabinoid, anandamide, seems particularly important, as it helps to regulate the activity of our amygdala—a brain region linked with anxiety. By regulating the activity in this part of our brain, anandamide can contribute to lower feelings of anxiety post-run (Heijnen et al., 2016).

There are also several psychological mechanisms to explain how running helps us feel better. Running can provide a time-out that helps to take our mind off stressors and worries in our life. Findings that distraction during running is linked with better mood after exercise, and that exercise in nature settings helps to reduce rumination (constant, repetitive thoughts about a problem), provides some support for this distraction hypothesis (Bratman et al., 2015). As we highlighted in the previous sections of this chapter, long-term running can also provide a sense of achievement when we run further or faster, increase our fitness, or accomplish our goals. In turn, this sense of achievement helps to increase self-esteem and boost our self-concept—that is how we perceive various characteristics of ourselves (like "I am good at running" or "I work hard to achieve my goals"). In turn, higher self-esteem and self-concept are associated with lower symptoms of mental health conditions, such as anxiety.

Specific to anxiety and depression, running can also increase both feelings of energy/activation and feelings of pleasure, as explained in the *Affective States* section in Chapter 2. Anxiety disorders are characterised by feelings of tension and distress that, in terms of affective states, reflect high activation that feels unpleasant. Depressive disorders, in contrast, are characterised by feelings such as fatigue and low mood that, in terms of affective states, reflect low activation that feels unpleasant. One theory, called the Core Affect Hypothesis explains that increasing both activation (for example, feeling more energised) and feelings of pleasure (for example, feeling more excitement) through activities like running can be helpful to relieve symptoms of depression, whereas an increase in feelings of pleasure (for example, feeling more relaxed, calmer) can help to relieve symptoms of anxiety (Rebar et al., 2015). Together, these changes can help to boost our mood, lower symptoms of anxiety and depression, and help us feel better after running.

Finally, running can also expose us to many symptoms of anxiety, like a rapid heart rate and faster breathing, and teach us that these are normal responses that can be tolerated and do not need to be avoided. In turn, this can help people with an anxiety disorder to unlearn links between physical symptoms of anxiety and the causes of their anxiety, such as social situations, and to better understand and control their symptoms as a result (Herring et al., 2014).

RUNNING AND BRAIN HEALTH

Running can also have multiple benefits for the structure and function of our brain. We each have a myriad of mental abilities, known as *cognitive functions*, and these functions include attention (such as our ability to concentrate or to shift our focus between tasks), perception (such as recognising, interpreting, and responding to information around us, such as objects or sounds), language (such as reading, writing, comprehension, naming people or objects), and long-term memory (such as remembering facts, life events, or how to do things). Cognitive functions also include a range of mental processes called *executive functions*, which include working memory (such as performing math in your head or translating instructions, like directions, into action plans), planning, decision-making, problem-solving, and inhibitory control (such as overriding various impulses or habits in favour of more appropriate responses, such as not eating cake when dieting or keeping going despite urges to stop during a run). Researchers typically use a range of different tasks to test each of these cognitive functions and you can find examples of these experiments—and test your own cognitive functions—by exploring the library of experiments at www.psytoolkit.org/. We came across one of these tasks, the Stroop task, in Chapter 2 when we explored the effects of mental fatigue on running performance. In this section, we will provide an insight into the effects of aerobic exercise, including walking, running, and cycling, on cognitive function.

A single bout of aerobic exercise can lead to small improvements in many cognitive functions in both children and adults that can last for up to two hours post-activity. These improvements are primarily for tasks that depend on a region of our brain called the prefrontal cortex. Benefits include an increased ability to focus attention and improvements in many executive functions like working memory, problem solving, decision-making, and verbal fluency (tasks such as naming as many animals as possible in 60 seconds). Some evidence also points to an impact on other areas of our brain and functions associated with these areas. These include improvements in longer-term memory associated with a region of the brain called the hippocampus, and improvements in learning and retention of information associated with a region of the brain called the striatum (Basso & Suzuki, 2017). The improvements in brain function after a bout of running also depend on the duration and intensity of our activity, however. At least ten to 20 minutes of aerobic activity is necessary to improve cognitive function, and low- or moderate-intensity activity leads to positive effects immediately after exercise. On the other hand, longer-duration activity, such as running for two hours or more, can lead to worse cognitive function, most likely because of fatigue and dehydration. Similarly, hard or very hard exercise results in worse mental performance in the first few minutes after activity (try to calculate 93 X 7 immediately on crossing the finish line after a maximum effort 5km!) but boosts cognitive function after this initial post-exercise period (Chang et al., 2012).

Longer-term aerobic exercise also leads to more lasting changes in brain structure and function. In children, longer-term activity can improve many of the cognitive functions highlighted earlier (Tomporowski et al., 2015). In one study, overweight children aged between seven and 11 years old who completed 13 weeks of vigorous-intensity activity showed improvements in executive functions, like their ability to plan, but not in other cognitive functions, like attention. The children completed the exercise sessions five days per week and completed either 20 minutes or 40 minutes of running games, rope jumping, or modified basketball and soccer games. Those who completed more activity demonstrated greater improvements in executive functions and also improvements on a test of mathematics achievement (Davis et al., 2011). In young and middle-aged adults, longer-term activity has also been shown to improve executive functions and memory (Cox et al., 2016). In older adults, such as those aged 55 years and above, longer-term aerobic exercise leads to improvements in brain functions such as attention, memory, and executive functions, like planning and problem-solving. In one study, 24 previously inactive 70-year-olds completed either 12 weeks of aerobic activity or a stretching programme. The aerobic activity consisted of 40 minutes of moderate-intensity walking and circuit training that gradually increased to a running intensity. After the 12 weeks, people in the aerobic training group improved their performance in a cognitive task called the Wisconsin Card Sorting Task, a test of executive functions including working memory and inhibition functions that are particularly vulnerable to decline as we grow older (Albinet et al., 2010). No such improvements occurred in the stretching group.

Many of these improvements in brain function are underpinned by changes in the structure of the same brain regions that are influenced by a single bout of running. These changes include increases in the volume of the outer part of our brain, called the cerebral cortex, including in specific areas called the frontal, parietal, and temporal regions. These areas of our brain are important for working memory, attention, and concentration; for performing executive functions like problem-solving; for engaging in tasks like reading and mathematics; and for our ability to recognise people or objects. Aerobic exercise also leads to an increase in the volume of the hippocampus—a part of our brain associated with memory. By increasing the volume of this brain region, exercise can help to reverse some of the declines in brain structure and functions like memory that we experience as we get older. Importantly, these changes in brain structure and function result from prolonged aerobic activity, or from aerobic exercise in combination with resistance training, but not when we only perform very low-intensity activities, like light stretching (Kramer & Colcombe, 2018). Taken as a whole, these findings show that running impacts multiple brain functions and results in a healthier, more efficient, and better-performing brain across our lifespan.

How and why this happens can be explained, in part, by the Adaptive Capacity Model that we introduced in Chapter 1 (Raichlen & Alexander, 2017). Just like a muscle will adapt to exercise, our brain also adapts to physically and mentally challenging activities, like running. More so, running in an environment that provides greater mental challenges, such as navigating your way on an outdoor trail or path, might provide an additional stimulus to boost the health of your brain. The trigger for these improvements—exercise—increases blood flow to our brain. Longer-term exercise also results in the growth in new blood vessels that supply oxygen and nutrient-rich blood to different regions of our brain (Fabel et al., 2003). Exercise also leads to the production of *neurotrophins*, a family of proteins that, when produced, impact the structure of nerve cells in our body. One neurotrophin, brain-derived neurotrophic factor (BDNF), leads to the formation of new brain cells in a process called neurogenesis (Cotman & Berchtold, 2002). In turn, these new cells, and greater interconnectivity between existing brain cells, can lead to many of the improvements in brain function outlined in this section.

Given the positive impact of running on both our mental health and brain health outlined in this chapter, it seems that running can do no wrong. But is this true? Can running also have a darker side? To provide a fully balanced answer to the question, "Can running help me feel better?", it is important to highlight that, despite these many benefits, in some circumstances, running can also have a downside.

EXERCISE ADDICTION: THE DARK SIDE OF RUNNING

Because of the benefits associated with exercise, many people are highly committed to running, and derive enjoyment, satisfaction, and a sense of achievement from training and racing. For many, running is a form of therapy. A separate phenomenon, distinct from this commitment, however, is *exercise addiction*. There are many terms used to describe exercise addiction, such as exercise dependence, exercise abuse, or obligatory exercise, but the concept was introduced in the early 1980s as *running addiction* to describe withdrawal symptoms, like anxiety and tension, that were experienced when committed runners were unable to run (Sachs & Pargman, 1984). In this section, we will mostly refer to exercise addiction, but we will also present some studies that have measured exercise dependence. A key difference between these two terms is that addiction incorporates both a dependence and a compulsion to engage in exercise behaviour.

Exercise addiction is a psychological condition linked to over-exercising. For committed runners, running is an important part of their lives, but it is not the most important aspect, and committed runners do not tend to experience withdrawal symptoms when they cannot run. In contrast, for those with exercise addiction, exercise is the central and most important part of their lives, and they often experience withdrawal as one of a range of symptoms when prevented from exercising for some reason. The incentives to exercise are also different between a committed exerciser and someone with exercise addiction. While a committed exerciser might be motivated by the positive aspects of an activity and gaining some feeling of reward from taking part (for example, to feel good afterwards, to be with friends, to stay fit and healthy, to accomplish something like finishing a 5km run), those with exercise addiction are often motivated to exercise both by these positive aspects *and* to avoid something negative or unpleasant. These negative aspects might be experiencing withdrawal symptoms, being unable to cope with stress in their lives, or feeling like they are getting fat by missing an exercise session. In this way, participation in exercise can often begin as something positive that a person *wants to do* for the benefits associated with it. However, each time we exercise to avoid something negative, these alternative motives are strengthened. Over time, exercise is driven more by the prevention and avoidance of something negative and, consequently, something the person feels they *have to do* on a regular basis (Szabo & Egorov, 2016). Exactly when, why, or how this transition takes place is not well understood.

Exercise addiction can be classified as primary exercise addiction and secondary exercise addiction. In secondary exercise addiction, the addiction is present alongside an eating disorder, and both exercise and disordered eating are used for the specific purpose of weight loss. As such, the mechanism leading to secondary exercise addiction—where the objective is to lose weight—is different from those of primary exercise addiction, where exercising in and of itself is the objective. The focus in this section is on primary exercise addiction. In total, there are six symptoms of exercise addiction, each relevant to runners. Each of these symptoms are important to diagnose exercise addiction and, unlike the early work that highlighted withdrawal symptoms only, we now understand that no single symptom alone implies an addiction to exercise. Considering the range of symptoms and the intensity of each is important, and later in this section we will outline how to assess risk of exercise addiction.

The first symptom of exercise addiction is *salience*, a symptom that is present when exercise dominates our thinking, feelings (cravings), and behaviour. Exercise becomes the most important activity in a person's life and is always on their mind, regardless of other activities, such as social engagements or work, that they might be engaged in at the time. Second is *conflict*, whereby the time or thought devoted to exercise means that relationships with family or friends are neglected, exercise is prioritised over work activities or other interests, or the person experiences an internal conflict where they realise that exercise dominates their life, but they are still unable to reduce or control exercising despite this awareness. Third is *mood modification*, where the person feels good or experiences a high after exercise. While this is a benefit for many exercisers, and a positive effect of running highlighted in this chapter, for those with exercise addiction, the motive is not only to feel good, but also to avoid the negative feelings, like low mood or guilt, that they would experience if they did not exercise. Fourth is *tolerance*, whereby progressively greater amounts of exercise are needed to experience the same effects, such as mood improvements, previously experienced with lesser amounts of exercise. This means that those with exercise addiction often increase the frequency, duration, and intensity of sessions simply to experience the same effects that a lesser amount of exercise used to provide. Fifth is *withdrawal*, which is severe, unpleasant psychological or physical symptoms experienced when exercise is reduced or stopped. Withdrawal symptoms might include feeling irritable, guilty, anxious, miserable, or lacking energy. Importantly, for those with exercise addiction, there is a compulsion—a "*have to exercise*"—to overcome these symptoms. Finally, *relapse* is a return to previous levels of activity after a voluntary (for example, trying to stop) or an involuntary (for example, through injury) break from exercise. Relapse means that those with addiction often return to their previous levels of activity, or do even more than previously, after taking this break.

Amongst the general population, the number of people considered at-risk of exercise dependence and exercise addiction seems relatively low. While figures vary, studies using valid scales have reported that about 1% to 3% of the general exercising population are at-risk, rising to about 6% to 8% for regular gym users and sport students

(Griffiths et al., 2005; Mónok et al., 2012; Warner & Griffiths, 2006). In runners, some studies have reported much higher figures for risk of exercise dependence and exercise addiction, with figures ranging from 20% to 77% (McNamara & McCabe, 2013; Smith et al., 2010; Thornton & Scott, 1995). A large study amongst 1285 triathletes, for example, identified 20% were at-risk of exercise addiction, with those training for longer distances, such as for a Half Ironman and Ironman, at a higher risk than those training for shorter sprint events (Youngman & Simpson, 2014). In other studies, the figure reported is much lower, with 3.2% of a group of ultra-marathon runners screened as at-risk of exercise dependence, for example (Allegre et al., 2007). These ranges of figures highlight some of the issues in the study of exercise addiction and one of the reasons for these large variations is confusion about how exercise dependence and exercise addiction are defined. This confusion means that committed runners are sometimes incorrectly classified as runners at-risk of exercise dependence or addiction (more on this later). Despite this confusion, runners and those who take part in endurance events do seem to be at a higher risk of exercise dependence and exercise addiction than the general population.

There are many models that attempt to explain the psychological processes leading to exercise dependence and exercise addiction. The Cognitive Appraisal Hypothesis (Szabo, 1995), for example, highlights the impact of life-stress and explains that, for some, exercise is their primary means of coping with stress. As a result, they become dependent on exercise as a coping mechanism. If other life demands interfere with or reduce exercise time, then people lose their only coping mechanism and experience hardship and withdrawal symptoms as a result. While this model can account for the use of exercise as a means of coping, it does not explain how, or for whom, exercise addiction occurs to begin with.

A four-phase model (Freimuth et al., 2011) attempts to fill this gap and explains that recreational exercise begins as a pleasurable and rewarding activity for many people. This is phase one. In phase two, the ability of exercise to boost mood is recognised by the person and exercise is used to help cope with difficult moments in their life. In this phase, individuals are now at-risk of developing exercise addiction. While some might have other means of coping with stress, for others, exercise becomes their sole coping mechanism, though why this happens is unclear in this model. In phase three, exercise becomes problematic and daily life is organised around exercise to the exclusion of other activities, like time with friends and family, leading to negative consequences like conflict with partners and feelings of withdrawal if exercise is reduced. At this point, maintaining control over exercising becomes difficult. In the final phase, exercise addiction fully manifests, and all six symptoms of exercise addiction are present.

What ultimately determines who might experience an addiction to exercise is highlighted in a final, *interactional model* (Egorov & Szabo, 2013). This model suggests that multiple personal factors (for example, personality, interests and goals, personal needs and values), situational factors (for example, accessibility and cost of exercise, social aspects of someone's life), and exercise motivations (for example, for health, performance, or social aspects) can all interact to determine who might gravitate toward using exercise as a means of coping when a sudden or intolerable life-stress is experienced. While the many possible interactions between each of these factors make it virtually impossible to predict who might experience exercise addiction, this model does help us identify the underlying causes that can lead to exercise addiction and help treat exercise addiction when it occurs. In research with runners, the importance of some of these factors are highlighted by individual studies. Specific predictors of being at-risk of exercise dependence or addiction in runners include having a stronger identity as a runner, being motivated to run mostly to avoid feelings of guilt or anxiety, the number of runs completed per week, weekly training hours, and the number of times injured in the previous two years (Hamer et al., 2002; Maceri et al., 2021). Amongst ultra-marathon runners, younger age, lower body mass index (lower body mass relative to height), higher total physical activity, but with less-moderate intensity physical activity, all predicted higher risk of exercise dependence (Allegre et al., 2007). These findings help to highlight some factors that might predict our risk of exercise addiction. In the *Run With It* section of this chapter, we have provided a tool that you can use to screen for your risk of exercise addiction, and some advice to follow if you are concerned.

KEY POINTS ON RUNNING, MENTAL HEALTH, AND BRAIN HEALTH

1. A single bout of running can boost our mood and improve how we feel. Maximum benefits come from no more than 40 minutes at a comfortable pace or 20–30 minutes at a harder pace. Running in nature can add to these benefits.

2. Weeks and months of regular running lead to longer-term benefits such as improved mood, higher psychological wellbeing, and lower anxiety and depression. To maximise benefits, running for three or more times per week is best, though any running is better than none. Doing some weekly runs with friends can add to these benefits.

3. There are many biological and psychological mechanisms to explain why running changes how we feel. Running can boost feel-good chemicals in our brain, like serotonin and dopamine. Running can also provide a distraction from daily worries, help to build our self-esteem, and increase feelings of energy and pleasure.

4. Running can also improve the health of our brain. A single bout of running can improve concentration, enhance memory, and augment our abilities to solve problems and make decisions after running. Longer-term running can improve brain structure and function throughout our lifespan and delay or reverse age-related decline in attention, memory, and mental abilities, like planning and problem solving.

5. The beneficial effects of running can lead to exercise addiction in some. There are six symptoms of exercise addiction: salience, conflict, mood modification, tolerance, withdrawal, and relapse.

If you are concerned about these symptoms or feel that you might be at-risk, consider contacting a health professional for advice.

RUN WITH IT: HOW CAN I SCREEN MY RISK FOR EXERCISE ADDICTION?

In this chapter, we highlighted a downside to running: Exercise addiction. This might lead to an important question for you: How can I screen my risk of exercise addiction? Several scales have been developed since the early 1980s to assess exercise dependence and exercise addiction. To highlight why some confusion exists in this area, one example, the Running Addiction Scale (Chapman & De Castro, 1990) includes items such as, "*I run on a regular basis,*" "*If the weather is too cold, too hot, or too windy, I will not run that day,*" and "*After I run I feel better*" that do not distinguish a committed runner from a runner at risk of a running addiction.

More recent scales provide a better measure of the risk of exercise addiction. One short, freely available scale to screen for the risk of exercise addiction is the Exercise Addiction Inventory (EAI: Terry et al., 2004). A version of the EAI is included below and this scale has been used in some recent studies to identify risk of exercise addiction in runners. It contains six items, each rated on a five-point scale from 1 (*Strongly Disagree*) to 5 (*Strongly Agree*), and items relate to symptoms of addiction, namely salience, conflict, mood modification, tolerance, withdrawal, and relapse. A total score of 24 or higher on the EAI indicates a risk of exercise addiction. It's important to note that this is a screening tool, and even someone scoring 24 or higher may not necessarily be experiencing an addiction to exercise, but instead is considered *at-risk* of exercise addiction.

If you are concerned by your score on the EAI, you should contact a health professional who may refer you to a qualified psychologist or psychiatrist who specialises in treating addictions. They will perform an in-depth interview to first diagnose exercise addiction before working to identify and treat the causes of exercise addition using appropriate therapeutic interventions. These interventions might

Table 5.2 Exercise Addiction Inventory (EAI; Terry et al., 2004). Circle your response for each item (from 1 to 5) and sum your responses for a total score on the EAI. A total score of 24 or higher indicates someone is "at-risk" from exercise addiction.

	Strongly Disagree	Disagree	Neither Agree nor Disagree	Agree	Strongly Agree
Exercise is the most important thing in my life	1	2	3	4	5
Conflicts have arisen between me and my family and/or my partner about the amount of exercise I do	1	2	3	4	5
I use exercise as a way of changing my mood (such as to get a buzz, to escape)	1	2	3	4	5
Over time I have increased the amount of exercise I do in a day	1	2	3	4	5
If I have to miss an exercise session, I feel moody and irritable	1	2	3	4	5
If I cut down the amount of exercise I do, and then start again, I always end up exercising as often as I did before	1	2	3	4	5
Total Score for the EAI (Sum of scores for all six items)					

include education on exercise addiction and the underlying causes, recommendations on how to reduce and control exercise behaviours, work to develop other coping strategies to deal with stress, or help to challenge and modify unhelpful thoughts that can drive compulsive exercise behaviours. The ultimate goal is to help people experiencing exercise addiction to achieve greater balance in their lives and regain control over their exercise behaviours.

6

ARE RUNNING-BASED PROGRAMMES BENEFICIAL FOR CHILDREN AND ADULTS?

INTRODUCTION

Around the world, there are school- and community-based programmes that can accommodate the running needs of everyone. The
programmes that we will present in this chapter all have different
aims and target different groups, but each have running at the core of
the services they provide. Beginning in primary school (ages four to
11), The Daily Mile was initiated in Scotland to provide children with
a 15-minute bout of physical activity on at least three days per week.
Since beginning in 2012, The Daily Mile now involves approximately
4 million children across 90 different countries on a weekly basis. In
the United States and Canada, Girls on the Run provides schoolgirls
aged 8–14 years with a ten-week running programme that serves as
a vehicle to develop life skills, such as skills to help regulate emotions
and resolve conflicts with others. Since the first Girls on the Run event
in 1996, over 2.25 million girls across 170 different locations in the
U.S.A. and Canada have completed the programme.

For older children and adults, parkrun is a free, timed 5km walking or running event that takes place every weekend in approximately
2,200 locations across 22 different countries. Since the first event in

DOI: 10.4324/9781003204206-7

2004, over 4 million people have taken part in parkrun worldwide. To provide greater opportunities for younger children to increase their activity levels, junior parkrun was established in 2013 to provide a weekly 2km running event for 4–14-year-olds. Finally, running charities also exist that use running as a platform to help those experiencing homelessness or are at risk of homelessness. These include The Running Charity and A Mile in Her Shoes in the U.K., and Back on My Feet in the U.S.A. In this chapter, we will explore each of these school- and community-based programmes, and explore the physical, mental, and social health benefits associated with each, beginning with The Daily Mile.

THE DAILY MILE

The Daily Mile is a primary school-based initiative that aims to provide children with a 15-minute bout of running, walking, or wheeling on a minimum of three days per week. The 15-minute period of activity amounts to about one mile of distance covered, hence The Daily Mile name. The initiative started in St Ninian's Primary School in Stirling, Scotland, in 2012 when headteacher Elaine Wyllie grew concerned about the lack of fitness displayed by the school's children. As a response to these concerns, she encouraged the children to run around the school's playground for 15 minutes during each school day. Soon, the entire school was participating in the daily activity, and it's reported that not one of the school's 57 children were deemed overweight by the school's nurse by the end of that year (see The Daily Mile website at www.thedailymile.org).

From these early beginnings, The Daily Mile has grown and spread to schools around the world. At the time of writing, almost 4 million children in more than 16,000 schools within 90 countries are registered to complete The Daily Mile. Practice of The Daily Mile is shaped around 10 core principles. These are that The Daily Mile should be quick and simple, taking just 15 minutes to complete with no time spent changing into a special kit, setting up, or tidying up. It should be fun, allowing children to chat with their friends as they participate, and should be fully inclusive, meaning that every child should be supported to take part every day. The Daily Mile should take place regardless of the weather, on a safe route and on a firm, mud-free surface. The Daily Mile should happen during the school day at least three times a week and should not replace physical education classes. Children are encouraged to go at their own pace, though the aim is to run, jog, or wheel for the full 15 minutes with only occasional stops to catch their breath.

To explore the effects of The Daily Mile on children's health, we (Breslin et al., 2023) completed a review of the effects of The Daily Mile on children's physical activity levels and on their physical health, mental health, academic performance, and on cognitive functions such as attention and memory. Perhaps not surprisingly, we found that The Daily Mile led to significantly higher physical activity levels in school children. Those that completed The Daily Mile achieved about 10 additional minutes per day of moderate-to-vigorous-intensity physical activity—an intensity that is linked with improved health benefits for children, such as lower body fatness and improved blood pressure and metabolic health. This increased activity led to significant gains in physical fitness and improvements in body composition (that is, reductions in body fat) in some, but not all studies. Improvements in body composition were largest for those who completed the activity on three or more days per week.

In terms of The Daily Mile's impact on children's mental health, in one study, parents of 550 children aged 5–13 years reported reductions in total difficulties experienced by their child, including lower hyperactivity (that is, children were less restless and better able to stay still for a long period), fewer problems interacting with other children, the children were more helpful and more considerate of other people's feelings, and experienced fewer emotional problems, such as fewer worries or felt less nervous in new situations (Arkesteyn et al., 2022). The same study also reported increases in children's feelings of self-worth and self-esteem, particularly for children with low feelings of self-worth and self-esteem to begin with. Specifically, these children reported increases in how competent they felt about doing schoolwork, how popular or accepted they felt about social interactions with their peers, and how competent they felt at doing sports and games requiring physical or athletic ability. These children also felt better about the way they behaved and about their overall physical appearance. These changes were noted after ten to 20 weeks of participation in The Daily Mile.

A single bout of The Daily Mile did not appear to have any effects on measures of academic performance. One study did report that three months or more of The Daily Mile led to higher scores on a test of visual spatial working memory, which involves our ability to recall shapes, colours, and their locations—important abilities that underpin our reading and writing skills, for example (Booth et al., 2022). Another study found that five weeks of The Daily Mile led to improvements in children's attention and short-term working memory (Dring et al., 2022).

Overall, while there is some evidence to suggest that longer-term participation in The Daily Mile can improve children's physical fitness, mental health, and some cognitive functions, our review highlighted a need for high-quality studies on the impact of The Daily Mile on children's physical and mental health. New research is ongoing, however, and one study, called the iMprOVE trial, that might shed greater light on the impact of The Daily Mile on primary-school children's physical and mental health and educational attainment, is currently underway in primary schools in Greater London (Ram et al., 2021). That study aims to recruit over 3,500 children, half of which complete The Daily Mile and half who don't, to track their health and educational outcomes throughout their primary school years. The first complete set of results for this study are due in 2026, which should give some insight into the longer-term effects of The Daily Mile on children's physical health, mental health, and educational attainment.

GIRLS ON THE RUN

While The Daily Mile predominantly focuses on increasing children's physical activity levels, some programmes exist that promote life-skill development in children alongside weekly physical activity. These include Let me Run, which aims to help boys get more active, learn teamwork, build relationship skills, create friendships, and develop emotionally (www.letmerun.org). Let me Run started in 2008 by Ashley Arimstead, who had served as a volunteer coach of a separate programme specifically aimed at girls, called Girls on the Run. Founded in 1996 in Charlotte, North Carolina, by Molly Barker, Girls on the Run is an after-school positive youth development programme that uses physical activity as a vehicle to develop life skills among girls (www.girlsontherun.org). Over a period of ten weeks, the programme combines training for a 5km event with twice-weekly curriculum-based activities that are organised around a five Cs framework of positive youth development (Lerner et al., 2005). Specifically, the 75- to 90-minute lessons are designed to help girls develop physical, emotional, and social *competence* (for example, feel better at doing physical activities, improve their ability to regulate emotions, find it easier to make friends), to feel more *confident* (for example, about how one looks), to create positive *connections* with others (for example, feel that others like them the way they are), to develop *character* (for example, to respect, help, or be kind to others), and to respond to others and oneself with *care* and compassion (for example, feel empathy for others). A sixth C, *contribution*, is also developed through taking part in a separate community service project, such as supporting people with an illness, collecting donations for animal shelters, or helping to improve the environment by cleaning up their school and community (Weiss et al., 2019). Despite the name, Girls on the Run is inclusive of activities other than running, and girls can walk, wheel, or engage in any other movement during the ten-week programme.

There are two separate programmes within Girls on the Run. First is a third to fifth grade (age 8–11 years) programme, also called Girls on the Run, that focuses on three main themes: identity (understanding oneself and developing self-care skills), connectedness (developing and valuing healthy relationships), and empowerment (celebrating and sharing one's strengths). Second is a sixth to eighth grade (age 12–14 years) programme called Heart & Sole that includes lessons emphasising the whole girl: her body, brain, heart, spirit, and social connections. Girls learn more about themselves, build inner strength, and become independent and critical thinkers. Training for a 5km event helps girls in both programmes to set, track, and achieve goals; to increase physical fitness; and to build confidence as they progress through the ten weeks of activities. To prepare specifically for the 5km event, girls learn to find their "feel good" pace and are encouraged to keep moving, regardless of whether they walk, run, wheel, skip, jump, or hop to the finish line. Girls are encouraged to embrace a philosophy of having fun and focus on their own effort and personal improvement instead of how they compare to others.

Some of the life skills developed through Girls on the Run incorporate psychological techniques that we introduced in Chapters 3 and 4 of this book. These include *Set Goals*, such as goals related to completing the 5km event or to improve academic performance in school, and *Star Power*, where girls learn how to use mental imagery to increase confidence to complete schoolwork, for example, or to imagine standing up for themselves with peers. The *Stop and take a BrThRR* strategy teaches girls to pause (that is, *Stop*), take a centering breath, think about the situation they are experiencing, respond in a constructive way, and subsequently review the effectiveness of their response. The aim is to help girls manage their emotions more effectively. Other strategies include *Change negative self-talk to positive self-talk*, which girls learn to apply both to running and life contexts to remain more positive in challenging situations, and *I feel . . . when you . . . because . . . and I would like for you to . . .*, which gives girls a framework to assertively express how they feel and resolve conflict with peers or family members (Weiss et al., 2020).

To date, more than 2.25 million girls have completed Girls on the Run, and many studies have explored the benefits of the programme. These studies have shown that, as well as increasing physical activity levels and reducing time spent watching TV and playing computer games, the programme helps to increase self-esteem (DeBate & Thompson, 2005; DeBate et al., 2009); improve perceptions of self-worth, physical appearance, body image, and social competence

(Pettee Gabriel et al., 2011; Sifers & Shea, 2013); and increases girls' physical self-concept (Martin et al., 2009). What these changes mean is that girls who completed Girls on the Run felt happier with themselves as a person and the way they looked, perceived that they were more skilled at making friends, and showed increases in physical activity and improvements in their overall physical health because of the ten-week programme.

Recently, more rigorous examinations of the programme led by professor Maureen Weiss have shown that girls' emotional, social, and physical behaviours improve because of participation in the programme especially for those with lower scores to begin with (Weiss et al., 2020). In line with the five Cs underpinning Girls on the Run, positive changes were noted for physical and social *competence* (for example, girls felt they were better at physical activities and at managing social interactions), feelings of *confidence* (for example, feeling more empowered or greater acceptance of oneself), feeling more *connected* (for example, improved friendships and being more accepting of others), and improved *character* and *caring* behaviours (for example, being kind to others or standing up for oneself and others).

The programme also helps to develop a healthier lifestyle in girls, characterised by positive changes in physical health (for example, staying fit, being more physically active), nutritional behaviours (for example, eating more fruit and vegetables and less junk food), emotional health (for example, being less impulsive, better able to control anger, reduced anxiety, improved ability to manage stress), mental health (for example, increased self-esteem through achieving running goals), and social health (for example, able to connect more with others, having a stronger core of friends) (Weiss et al., 2020). More so, a 2020 evaluation found that girls who completed the Girls on the Run programme reported stronger abilities to manage emotions (such as calm themselves when angry or frustrated), resolve conflicts (such as disagreements with family or friends), help or stand up for others, and make intentional decisions (such as think before acting) in other areas of their life outside of physical activity. These benefits endured three months after finishing the programme, suggesting that Girls on the Run has a longer-lasting impact, even after formal lessons have ended (Weiss et al., 2020).

PARKRUN

parkrun is a free, timed, community-based event that takes place weekly in public parks. It is open to people of all ages, abilities, and backgrounds to take part as walkers, joggers, runners, or as volunteers to help deliver each parkrun event. It began in 2004 in Bushy Park, London, when Paul Sinton-Hewitt initiated the Bushy Park Time Trial, a 5km event that started with just 13 participants toeing the line, supported by a team of five volunteers. Since those humble origins, parkrun has grown into something of a global phenomenon that now takes place every weekend in approximately 2,200 locations across 22 different countries (www.parkrun.com). In the U.K. alone, more than 2.7 million people have participated in parkrun across 775 event locations (www.parkrun.org.uk), whereas in Ireland, approximately 223,000 people have participated in at least one of the 106 event locations (www.parkrun.ie). Since 2013, parkrun has also provided a weekly 2km event for 4–14-year-olds called junior parkrun, and more than 435,000 children have since participated in one of the 382 junior parkrun event locations in the U.K.

The popularity of parkrun is in part explained by the fact that it's free, open to people of all ages and abilities, and, because it is not a race, can be completed as a run or walk. People take part or volunteer for many reasons, including to get some exercise, to improve their physical health, to maintain or improve fitness, to compete against other people or one's own previous times, to gain a sense of achievement, to meet and interact with people, and to have fun (Bowness et al., 2021). First-time participants often come along with friends or family members, but taking part fosters a sense of community and belonging, and these social ties help to maintain longer-term parkrun participation (Wiltshire et al., 2018). As a result of taking part, people also report improved confidence in running, more strongly identify as "runners," and often become involved in formal running groups outside of parkrun (Hindley, 2020).

Alongside these social benefits, parkrun also brings many physical and mental health benefits (Grunseit et al., 2020; Peterson et al., 2022). In terms of physical health, parkrun participation has been associated with improved physical fitness and small reductions in bodyweight (about 1 kg on average) over a 12-month period, with greater changes observed amongst more regular participants and those who were overweight or obese to begin with (Stevinson & Hickson, 2019). parkrun also helps to improve people's weekly physical activity levels, with one study reporting that new parkrunners' total physical activity levels and vigorous-intensity physical activity levels increased by 76.9 minutes and 20.8 minutes, respectively, after six months of parkrun involvement (Stevinson & Hickson, 2019). Importantly, even after 12 months, people whose physical activity levels were below the recommended guidelines pre-parkrun (that is, either 150 minutes of total activity or 75 minutes of vigorous-intensity activity) had higher total physical activity (increased by 194.2 minutes per week) and vigorous-intensity activity (increased by 60.2 minutes per week) because of their parkrun involvement. What this figure shows is that taking part in parkrun can help to significantly increase physical activity levels and help those below the recommended guidelines pre-parkrun to reach the recommended levels of activity required to improve physical health.

parkrun involvement is also associated with improved mental health and wellbeing outcomes (Dunne et al., 2021). Completing a single 5km parkrun event has been shown to lower feelings of stress; lower negative moods such as tension, depression, anger, and confusion; increase feelings of vigour; and improve self-esteem. Key predictors of positive changes in mood were gender (females reported greater improvement in mood than males), enjoyment of the event, and feeling more connected with nature (that is, having a greater appreciation for and understanding of our interconnectedness with nature and the importance of nature), whereas improved self-esteem was associated with greater event enjoyment and satisfaction with one's performance (Rogerson et al., 2016). Regular participation over one year has also been shown to lower feelings of stress, reduce risk for depression, and increase feelings of happiness (Stevinson & Hickson, 2019). Amongst people who currently or had previously experienced mental health difficulties and had participated as a walker, runner, or volunteer in at least 10 parkrun events, the benefits of taking part were reduced feelings of social isolation, lower anxiety, depression, and stress, and higher feelings of confidence. These mental health benefits were underpinned by three key elements associated with parkrun: gaining a sense of achievement from completing a parkrun event, a belief that parkrun was inclusive and for everyone, and being able to connect with others through parkrun participation (Morris & Scott, 2019).

Collectively, these social, physical, and mental health benefits go some way to explain why parkrun is increasingly being prescribed by health practitioners as an intervention to improve their patients' physical and mental health. In the U.K., the Royal College of General Practitioners and parkrun U.K. developed the parkrun Practice initiative in 2018 which aims to improve the health and wellbeing of patients and practice staff, to raise awareness of the services that practices provide, to develop local communities centred around wellness, and to support the growth of social prescribing activities that signpost patients to non-medical and social activities like parkrun in their local community. Since 2018, over 1,500 General Practices—approximately 16% of the U.K. total—have linked with their local parkrun event (Fleming et al., 2022). The benefits of parkrun for health conditions are highlighted by the fact that health-related motives, including to manage weight, to improve mental health, and to improve or manage a disability, were recently highlighted as important motives for taking part in parkrun, especially by slower runners and walkers at parkrun events (Haake et al., 2022). More so, the top five health conditions reported by participants in this survey were depression, arthritis, anxiety, asthma, and high blood pressure, whereas slower runners and walkers also reported obesity, chronic pain, and type 2 diabetes. These findings highlight the importance of free, accessible events like parkrun to support the health and wellbeing of local communities, especially for those attempting to use exercise to manage a health condition. One further example of this in practice is 5k Your Way Move Against Cancer (www.5kyourway.org), a community-based initiative organised by the Move Charity that encourages those living with and beyond cancer, and their friends, families, and those working in cancer services to walk, jog, run, volunteer, or support at their local parkrun event on the last Saturday of every month.

RUNNING PROGRAMMES FOR PEOPLE EXPERIENCING HOMELESSNESS

Several charities also exist that use running as a vehicle to help those experiencing homelessness. These include The Running Charity in the U.K. (www.therunnigcharity.org) and Back on My Feet (www.back onmyfeet.org) in the U.S.A. Back on My Feet is a community-based programme that recruits individuals at homeless or addiction and treatment facilities in the U.S.A. Back on My Feet started in Philadelphia in 2007, but now spans 17 cities across the U.S.A. In total, it is a four-to-six-month programme that works with those living in homeless shelters. When people first join Back on My Feet, they commit to organised group running sessions on three mornings per week and are also encouraged to participate in local running races. During the first 30 days of the running programme, individuals who maintain at least 90% attendance at the running sessions progress into a Next Steps phase. Next Steps provides members with job skills training, education on financial literacy (for example, creating a budget, managing debt, tracking spending), and financial support to remove barriers to employment and housing, such as support for job training, educational fees, and transportation expenses. The goal of Back on My Feet is to help people achieve self-sufficiency through running, education, and job skills training by ultimately gaining employment and housing through their participation in the programme.

One study has explored the psychological benefits of the running element of Back on My Feet (Inoue et al., 2013). Before and immediately after the first 30 days of running, participants were asked to rate their psychological connection with running, such as running enjoyment and their perceived self-sufficiency. Perceived self-sufficiency was measured through changes in self-esteem, self-confidence, motivation to live a healthy lifestyle, feeling more productive in their daily life, feeling more trusting of others, and feeling more excited about their future. The findings showed that after the first 30 days, participants who maintained their involvement and running activity (about 43% of the initial group) reported a greater psychological connection with running in that they found running enjoyable, that it became an important part of their daily life, and that participating in running was viewed as a positive expression of their identity. In turn, a greater psychological connection with running predicted increases in participants' perceptions that they could attain self-sufficiency. As such, greater connection with running helped to increase participants self-esteem, self-confidence, and motivation to live a healthy lifestyle, independent of any other part of the programme, highlighting the positive benefits of running for those who maintained the activity.

A similar group-based running programme for homeless women is called A Mile in Her Shoes (www.amileinhershoes.org.uk). A Mile in Her Shoes is a charity based in London (U.K.) and provides volunteer-led running groups for women defined as homeless, at risk of homelessness, or affected by issues related to homelessness. The aim of A Mile in Her Shoes is to identify and remove barriers to running by providing suitable running clothing and access to women-only running groups, enabling participants to gain the physical, mental, and social health benefits associated with running. One interview-based study found that women who participated in the programme reported feeling a sense of achievement and purpose, and greater empowerment to cope with the challenging circumstances in their lives (Dawes et al., 2019). Although there were barriers to taking part in the programme, such as motivation, the unpredictability of being homeless, and feeling self-conscious when running, running also led to physical and mental health benefits for participants.

More so, participants reported feeling improved fitness and greater energy. In terms of mental health, participants also reported feeling higher confidence and improved mood, feeling happier and more relaxed, and feeling less lonely. In particular, the running programme also helped women to meet new people, make friends, and experience greater support from other women who had similar personal experiences to themselves.

Together, these studies give valuable insights into the value of group-based running programmes, such as Back on My Feet and A Mile in Her Shoes for those experiencing homelessness or at risk of homelessness. These programmes can provide many physical, mental, and social health benefits for some of the most vulnerable people in our society, helping to build self-esteem and self-confidence, and reduce feelings of loneliness.

KEY POINTS ABOUT SCHOOL- AND COMMUNITY-BASED PROGRAMMES

1. As little as 15 minutes of running per day, three times per week via The Daily Mile, improves body composition and increases feelings of self-worth and self-esteem in school children. Regularly taking part in The Daily Mile can also improve children's attention and short-term memory.
2. Running as part of a larger life-skills development programme, such as Girls on The Run, can help girls feel more competent, confident, connected with friends, and build their character and caring behaviours. Regular participation can also lead to a healthier lifestyle overall.
3. parkrun leads to many physical, mental, and social health benefits. In terms of mental health, parkrun helps to lower stress, lower risk of anxiety and depression, boost mood, increase feelings of happiness, and improve self-esteem.
4. Running charities that help those experiencing homelessness, like Back on My Feet and A Mile in Her Shoes, can increase self-esteem and self-confidence, reduce feelings of loneliness, and empower

people to cope with the challenging circumstances in their lives.

RUN WITH IT: GIRLS ON THE RUN

Research on Girls on the Run has highlighted the short- and long-term benefits of the programme for girl's physical, social, and emotional development. To learn a little more about the programme and to explore some longer-term benefits for those who take part, we spoke to two Girls on the Run alumni, Beth Gordon and Dillon McClintock.

Beth is a resident physician in internal medicine at New York University. She started as a participant in Girls on the Run in 2000 and completed the programme multiple times in both elementary school and in middle school. In college, she volunteered as a coach in the programme and has helped to train future Girls on the Run coaches in this role. Beth has continued to run since first completing the programme, running cross-country in middle school and high school, and has also completed a number of marathons.

Beth explained that participants in the programme can take whatever they feel helps them most in their life, whether that is the life-skills component, the running/physical activity component, or a combination of both.

> The whole premise was that you were building toward a 5k, but with every running exercise there was a life skills component, like communicating effectively, social negotiation, being true to yourself, or healthy lifestyles. There was a topic for every lesson, and then an exercise revolving around running but related to that lesson. So, for instance, one lesson was on how to articulate an emotion to someone else that might be uncomfortable. We'd first do a warm-up, then sit down and go through that lesson, and then do some activities that were running-related. So, you might first get a scenario on a card, do some running and formulate a response as you ran, and then practice how you might express that emotion to someone else. Some of the activities included

role play, some were naming emotions to develop a vocabulary for different emotions and articulating these, and sometimes it was funny things, like running while acting out that emotion for a lap.

Beth elaborated on how the lessons learned during Girls on the Run have helped her throughout her life since taking part in the programme.

While tailored to elementary or middle school girls, I think most of the lessons, like learning to feel confident with who you are, learning how to navigate relationships, or learning to take a second to think about what you want to say and how you want to say it, are all incredibly transferable life skills. There are still lessons that I'm working on now, however many years later. The programme aligns learning those life skills with something very physical. I feel that running is active meditation and I think that pairs nicely with some of the lessons that Girls on the Run includes. I still use running as a way to help sort stuff out and I wouldn't have known running could be that outlet for me if it wasn't for Girls on the Run.

One particularly impactful life skill component was a reflection on:

expectations of what a girl is, who a girl is, how she acts, and how she is in the world. We learned to question those expectations and whether those expectations are reasonable. We learned that you don't have to be perfect to move around in the world and that you don't have to meet everyone's expectations. We also learned to do things that are important to you and to separate that people-pleaser from who you are and what you want to do. I think that's a life skill that I still use to navigate the trickiness of expectations that are placed on you.

Dillon McClintock is a PhD student in mechanical engineering and, specifically, in soft tissue mechanics, at Michigan State University.

She first completed Girls on the Run in elementary school in 2008 and has volunteered in the programme multiple times since. Dillon continued her running career after Girls on the Run and competed as a middle-distance runner through middle school and high school, and at the collegiate level for Michigan State University. We asked Dillon why Girls on the Run is so popular, despite the fact that physical activities, like running, are not always easy to do.

> I feel that the unique thing about Girls on the Run versus team sports or other activities that you can do as a kid is that it does a really good job coupling doing hard things with making it fun and learning important lessons. With how it's structured, you don't just spend the entire time running as hard as you possibly can. It's not like a collegiate-level training regimen. It makes you *want* to be physically active, especially because it works on that goal setting aspect of working toward running a 5k at the end of the season and having an idea in your mind of what you're trying to reach. Plus, the fact that it's fun and you're doing it with your friends.
>
> The lessons are also integrated into the physical activity and that makes it easier to pay attention, especially for me, someone who's mind is moving at a million miles a minute. It makes it a lot easier to pay attention to the lesson because you're moving in between it and you're moving during the lesson. So, it's not just physically challenging, but it's mentally challenging too because you have to think about things. Because of that, I feel that it's an easy thing to want to be part of. It's an enjoyable activity!

The fun aspect and inclusivity of Girls on the Run is further reinforced during the final 5k. Dillon explained that:

> You can get through it whatever way you want. Some people walk it and some take it really seriously and run it fast. Because there are people stationed throughout the 5k course cheering on

with signs, sometimes kids will, literally, do cartwheels because they are excited that people are cheering them on. So, it's however you want to do it; you get from start to finish and you have completed your goal. From that aspect, it's really inclusive and it doesn't have to be an extremely competitive thing. It's more so just about completing that goal.

For Dillon, the lessons and life skills learned through Girls on the Run continued to help her throughout her running career. As a collegiate-level runner, lessons learned through Girls on the Run "gave me that confidence that I needed and the ability to trust myself that I am capable of doing what I'm attempting to do." These lessons continue to benefit Dillon now as she completes her PhD research in soft tissue mechanics.

A huge part of the programme is the confidence aspect and standing up for yourself and others. That has been a big thing for me. That also includes a lot of healthy relationship teachings too, like how to support healthy relationships and how to appropriately manage unhealthy relationships. That has helped me to manage in-group projects, like how to amplify the fact that I know how to do something. Even if I'm the only woman in the group and everyone else thinks they can do it, but I know for a fact that I can do it better because I did it in an internship or something. Or, like, standing up for myself when someone doesn't always want to listen to you. So, I feel from that standpoint, career-wise, it has definitely helped me a lot.

FURTHER READING

CHAPTER 1

Ogles, B. M., & Masters, K. S. (2003). A typology of marathon runners based on cluster analysis of motivations. *Journal of Sport Behavior, 26*(1), 69–85.

Raichlen, D. A., & Alexander, G. E. (2017). Adaptive capacity: An evolutionary neuroscience model linking exercise, cognition, and brain health. *Trends in Neurosciences, 40*(7), 408–421.

Roebuck, G. S., Fitzgerald, P. B., Urquhart, D. M., Ng, S. N., Cicuttini, F. M., & Fitzgibbon, B. M. (2018). The psychology of ultra-marathon runners: A systematic review. *Psychology of Sport and Exercise, 37*, 43–58.

CHAPTER 2

Anstiss, P. A., Meijen, C., & Marcora, S. M. (2020). The sources of self-efficacy in experienced and competitive endurance athletes. *International Journal of Sport and Exercise Psychology, 18*(5), 622–638.

Ekkekakis, P. (2003). Pleasure and displeasure from the body: Perspectives from exercise. *Cognition & Emotion, 17*(2), 213–239.

Marcora, S. (2019). Psychobiology of fatigue during endurance performance. In C. Meijen (Ed.), *Endurance performance in sport: Psychological theory and interventions* (pp. 15–34). Routledge.

Mauger, A. R. (2019). Exercise-induced pain: A psychophysiological perspective. In C. Meijen (Ed.), *Endurance performance in sport: Psychological theory and interventions* (pp. 35–46). Routledge.

Van Cutsem, J., Marcora, S., De Pauw, K., Bailey, S., Meeusen, R., & Roelands, B. (2017). The effects of mental fatigue on physical performance: A systematic review. *Sports Medicine, 47*(8), 1569–1588.

Venhorst, A., Micklewright, D., & Noakes, T. D. (2018a). Towards a three-dimensional framework of centrally regulated and goal-directed exercise behaviour: A narrative review. *British Journal of Sports Medicine, 52*(15), 957–966.

CHAPTER 3

Brick, N., MacIntyre, T., & Campbell, M. (2015). Metacognitive processes in the self-regulation of performance in elite endurance runners. *Psychology of Sport and Exercise, 19,* 1–9.

McCormick, A., Meijen, C., & Marcora, S. (2015). Psychological determinants of whole-body endurance performance. *Sports Medicine, 45,* 997–1015.

Williamson, O., Swann, C., Bennett, K. J. M., Bird, M. D., Goddard, S. G., Schweickle, M. J., & Jackman, P. C. (2022). The performance and psychological effects of goal setting in sport: A systematic review and meta-analysis. *International Review of Sport and Exercise Psychology,* Advance online publication.

CHAPTER 4

Brick, N., MacIntyre, T., & Campbell, M. (2014). Attentional focus in endurance activity: New paradigms and future directions. *International Review of Sport and Exercise Psychology, 7,* 106–134.

Corbally, L., Wilkinson, M., & Fothergill, M. A. (2020). Effects of mindfulness practice on performance and factors related to performance in long-distance running: A systematic review. *Journal of Clinical Sport Psychology, 14*(4), 376–398.

Karageorghis, C. I., & Priest, D. L. (2012a). Music in the exercise domain: A review and synthesis (Part I). *International Review of Sport and Exercise Psychology, 5*(1), 44–66.

Karageorghis, C. I., & Priest, D. L. (2012b). Music in the exercise domain: A review and synthesis (Part II). *International Review of Sport and Exercise Psychology, 5*(1), 67–84.

Terry, P. C., Karageorghis, C. I., Curran, M. L., Martin, O. V., & Parsons-Smith, R. L. (2020). Effects of music in exercise and sport: A meta-analytic review. *Psychological Bulletin, 146*(2), 91–117.

CHAPTER 5

Oswald, F., Campbell, J., Williamson, C., Richards, J., & Kelly, P. (2020). A scoping review of the relationship between running and mental health. *International Journal of Environmental Research and Public Health, 17*(21), 8059.

Reed, J., & Buck, S. (2009). The effect of regular aerobic exercise on positive-activated affect: A meta-analysis. *Psychology of Sport and Exercise, 10*(6), 581–594.

Reed, J., & Ones, D. S. (2006). The effect of acute aerobic exercise on positive activated affect: A meta-analysis. *Psychology of Sport and Exercise, 7*(5), 477–514.

Szabo, A., & Egorov, A. Y. (2016). Exercise addiction. In A. M. Lane (Ed.), *Sport and exercise psychology* (2nd ed., pp. 178–210). Routledge.

CHAPTER 6

Breslin, G., Hillyard, M., Brick, N., Shannon, S., McKay-Redmond, B., & McConnell, B. (2023). A systematic review of the effect of the daily mile on children's physical activity, physical health, mental health, wellbeing, academic performance and cognitive function, *PLoS One, 18*(1), e0277375.

Peterson, B., Withers, B., Hawke, F., Spink, M., Callister, R., & Chuter, V. (2022). Outcomes of participation in parkrun, and factors influencing why and how often individuals participate: A systematic review of quantitative studies. *Journal of Sports Sciences, 40*(13), 1486–1499.

Weiss, M. R., Kipp, L. E., Phillips Reichter, A., & Bolter, N. D. (2020). Evaluating girls on the run in promoting positive youth development: Group comparisons on life skills transfer and social processes. *Pediatric Exercise Science, 1*–11. Advance online publication.

Weiss, M. R., Kipp, L. E., Phillips Reichter, A., Espinoza, S. M., & Bolter, N. D. (2019). Girls on the run: Impact of a physical activity youth development program on psychosocial and behavioral outcomes. *Pediatric Exercise Science, 31*(3), 330–340.

REFERENCES

Achtziger, A., Gollwitzer, P. M., & Sheeran, P. (2008). Implementation intentions and shielding goal striving from unwanted thoughts and feelings. *Personality and Social Psychology Bulletin*, 34, 381–393.

Albinet, C. T., Boucard, G., Bouquet, C. A., & Audiffren, M. (2010). Increased heart rate variability and executive performance after aerobic training in the elderly. *European Journal of Applied Physiology*, 109, 617–624.

Allegre, B., Therme, P., & Griffiths, M. (2007). Individual factors and the context of physical activity in exercise dependence: A prospective study of "ultra-marathoners". *International Journal of Mental Health and Addiction*, 5(3), 233–243.

Alschuler, K. N., Krabak, B. J., Kratz, A. L., Jensen, M. P., Pomeranz, D., Burns, P., Bautz, J., Nordeen, C., Irwin, C., & Lipman, G. S. (2020). Pain is inevitable but suffering is optional: Relationship of pain coping strategies to performance in multistage ultramarathon runners. *Wilderness & Environmental Medicine*, 31(1), 23–30.

Anderson, J. J. (2021). *The state of running 2019*. https://runrepeat.com/state-of-running.

Anderson, R. J., & Brice, S. (2011). The mood-enhancing benefits of exercise: Memory biases augment the effect. *Psychology of Sport and Exercise*, 12(2), 79–82.

Anstiss, P. A., Meijen, C., Madigan, D. J., & Marcora, S. M. (2018). Development and initial validation of the endurance sport self-efficacy scale (ESSES). *Psychology of Sport and Exercise*, 38, 176–183.

Anstiss, P. A., Meijen, C., & Marcora, S. M. (2020). The sources of self-efficacy in experienced and competitive endurance athletes. *International Journal of Sport and Exercise Psychology*, 18(5), 622–638.

Antoniewicz, F., & Brand, R. (2016). Learning to like exercising: Evaluative conditioning changes automatic evaluations of exercising and influences subsequent exercising behavior. *Journal of Sport and Exercise Psychology*, 38(2), 138–148.

Arkesteyn, A., Van Campfort, D., Firth, J., & Van Damme, T. (2022). Mental health outcomes of the Daily Mile in elementary school children: A single-arm pilot study. *Child and Adolescent Mental Health*, 27(4), 361–368.

Balcetis, E., Riccio, M. T., Duncan, D. T., & Cole, S. (2020). Keeping the goal in sight: Testing the influence of narrowed visual attention on physical activity. *Personality and Social Psychology Bulletin*, 46(3), 485–496.

Ballmann, C. G. (2021). The influence of music preference on exercise responses and performance: A review. *Journal of Functional Morphology and Kinesiology*, 6(2), 33.

Barwood, M. J., Corbett, J., Wagstaff, C. R. D., McVeigh, D., & Thelwell, R. C. (2015). Improvement of 10-km time-trial cycling with motivational self-talk compared with neutral self-talk. *International Journal of Sports Physiology Performance*, 10, 166–171.

Barwood, M. J., Thelwell, R., & Tipton, M. (2008). Psychological skills training improves exercise performance in the heat. *Medicine and Science in Sports and Exercise*, 40(2), 398–406.

Basso, J. C., & Suzuki, W. A. (2017). The effects of acute exercise on mood, cognition, neurophysiology, and neurochemical pathways: A review. *Brain Plasticity (Amsterdam, Netherlands)*, 2(2), 127–152.

Bauman, A., Murphy, N., & Lane, A. (2009). The role of community programmes and mass events in promoting physical activity to patients. *British Journal of Sports Medicine*, 43(1), 44–46.

Berger, B. G., & Owen, D. R. (1998). Relation of low and moderate intensity exercise with acute mood change in college joggers. *Perceptual and Motor Skills*, 87(2), 611–621.

Bergevin, M., Steele, J., Payen de la Garanderie, M., Feral-Basin, C., Marcora, S. M., Rainville, P., Caron, J. G., & Pageaux, B. (2023). Pharmacological blockade of muscle afferents and perception of effort: A systematic review with meta-analysis. *Sports Medicine*, 53, 415–435.

Birrer, D., & Morgan, G. (2010). Psychological skill training as a way to enhance an athlete's performance in high-intensity sports. *Scandanavian Journal of Medicine and Science in Sports*, 20(2), 78–87.

Blanchfield, A. W., Hardy, J., de Morree, H. M., Staiano, W., & Marcora, S. M. (2014). Talking yourself out of exhaustion: The effects of self-talk on endurance performance. *Medicine and Science in Sports and Exercise*, 46, 998–1007.

Booth, J. N., Chesham, R. A., Brooks, N. E., Gorely, T., & Moran, C. N. (2022). The impact of The Daily Mile™ on school pupils' fitness, cognition, and wellbeing: Findings from longer term participation. *Frontiers in Psychology*, 13, 812616.

Borg, G. A. (1982). Psychophysical bases of perceived exertion. *Medicine and Science in Sports Exercise*, 14(5), 377–381.

Bowness, J., Tulle, E., & McKendrick, J. (2021). Understanding the parkrun community; sacred Saturdays and organic solidarity of park runners. *European Journal for Sport and Society*, 18(1), 44–63.

Bramble, D. M., & Lieberman, D. E. (2004). Endurance running and the evolution of *Homo*. *Nature*, 432, 345–352.

Bratman, G. N., Hamilton, J. P., Hahn, K. S., Daily, G. C., & Gross, J. J. (2015). Nature experience reduces rumination and subgenual prefrontal cortex activation. *PNAS*, 112, 8567–8572.

Brehm, J. W., & Self, E. A. (1989). The intensity of motivation. *Annual Review of Psychology*, 40(1), 109–131.

Breslin, G., Hillyard, M., Brick, N., Shannon, S., McKay-Redmond, B., & McConnell, B. (2023). A systematic review of the effect of The Daily Mile™ on children's physical activity, physical health, mental health, wellbeing, academic performance and cognitive function. *PLoS One*, 18(1), e0277375.

Brewer, B. W., Van Raalte, J. L., & Linder, D. E. (1996). Attentional focus and endurance performance. *Applied Research in Coaching and Athletics Annual*, 11, 1–14.

Brick, N. E., Campbell, M. J., Sheehan, R. B., Fitzpatrick, B. L., & MacIntyre, T. E. (2020). Metacognitive processes and attentional focus in recreational endurance runners. *International Journal of Sport and Exercise Psychology*, 18(3), 362–379.

Brick, N. E., Fitzpatrick, B. L., Turkington, R., & Mallett, J. C. (2019). Anticipated task difficulty provokes pace conservation and slower running performance. *Medicine and Science in Sports and Exercise*, 51(4), 734–743.

Brick, N. E., MacIntyre, T., & Campbell, M. (2014). Attentional focus in endurance activity: New paradigms and future directions. *International Review of Sport and Exercise Psychology*, 7, 106–134.

Brick, N. E., MacIntyre, T., & Campbell, M. (2015). Metacognitive processes in the self-regulation of performance in elite endurance runners. *Psychology of Sport and Exercise*, 19, 1–9.

Brick, N. E., McElhinney, M. J., & Metcalfe, R. S. (2018). The effects of facial expression and relaxation cues on movement economy, physiological, and perceptual responses during running. *Psychology of Sport and Exercise*, 34, 20–28.

Bueno, J., Weinberg, R. S., Fernández-Castro, J., & Capdevila, L. (2008). Emotional and motivational mechanisms mediating the influence of goal setting on endurance athletes' performance. *Psychology of Sport and Exercise*, 9(6), 786–799.

Burdina, M., Hiller, R. S., & Metz, N. E. (2017). Goal attainability and performance: Evidence from Boston marathon qualifying standards. *Journal of Economic Psychology*, 58, 77–88.

Burhans, R. S., Richman, C. L., & Bergey, D. B. (1988). Mental imagery training: Effects on running speed performance. *International Journal of Sport Psychology*, 19(1), 26–37.

Butryn, T. M., & Furst, D. M. (2003). The effects of park and urban settings on the moods and cognitive strategies of female runners. *Journal of Sport Behavior*, 26, 335–355.

Caird, S. J., McKenzie, A. D., & Sleivert, G. G. (1999). Biofeedback and relaxation techniques improve running economy in sub-elite long distance runners. *Medicine and Science in Sports and Exercise*, 31, 717–722.

Carrier, D. R. (1984). The energetic paradox of human running and hominid evolution. *Current Anthropology*, 25, 483–495.

Cerqueira, V., de Mendonça, A., Minez, A., Dias, A. R., & de Carvalho, M. (2006). Does caffeine modify corticomotor excitability? *Neurophysiologie Clinique/Clinical Neurophysiology*, 36(4), 219–226.

Chang, Y. K., Labban, J. D., Gapin, J. I., & Etnier, J. L. (2012). The effects of acute exercise on cognitive performance: A meta-analysis. *Brain Research*, 1453, 87–101.

Chapman, C. L., & De Castro, J. M. (1990). Running addiction: Measurement and associated psychological characteristics. *The Journal of Sports Medicine and Physical Fitness*, 30, 283–290.

Clarke, D. D., & Sokoloff, L. (1999). Regulation of cerebral metabolic rate. In G. J. Siegel, B. W. Agranoff, & R. W. Albers (Eds.), *Basic neurochemistry: Molecular, cellular and medical aspects*. Lippincott-Raven.

Colcombe, S. J., & Kramer, A. F. (2003). Fitness effects on the cognitive function of older adults: A meta-analytic study. *Psychological Science*, 14, 125–130.

Cole, S., Riccio, M., & Balcetis, E. (2014). Focused and fired up: Narrowed attention produces perceived proximity and increases goal-relevant action. *Motivation and Emotion*, 38, 815–822.

Cooper, K. B., Wilson, M. R., & Jones, M. I. (2021). Fast talkers? Investigating the influence of self-talk on mental toughness and finish times in 800-meter runners. *Journal of Applied Sport Psychology*, 33(5), 491–509.

Corbally, L., Wilkinson, M., & Fothergill, M. A. (2020). Effects of mindfulness practice on performance and factors related to performance in long-distance running: A systematic review. *Journal of Clinical Sport Psychology*, 14(4), 376–398.

Cotman, C. W., & Berchtold, N. C. (2002). Exercise: A behavioral intervention to enhance brain health and plasticity. *Trends in Neurosciences*, 25(6), 295–301.

Cox, E. P., O'Dwyer, N., Cook, R., Vetter, M., Cheng, H. L., Rooney, K., & O'Connor, H. (2016). Relationship between physical activity and cognitive function in apparently healthy young to middle-aged adults: A systematic review. *Journal of Science and Medicine in Sport*, 19(8), 616–628.

Davis, C. L., Tomporowski, P. D., McDowell, J. E., Austin, B. P., Miller, P. H., Yanasak, N. E., Allison, J. D., & Naglieri, J. A. (2011). Exercise improves executive function and achievement and alters brain activation in overweight children: A randomized, controlled trial. *Health Psychology*, 30(1), 91–98.

Dawes, J., Sanders, C., & Allen, R. (2019). "A mile in her shoes": A qualitative exploration of the perceived benefits of volunteer led running groups for homeless women. *Health & Social Care in the Community*, 27(5), 1232–1240.

DeBate, R. D., Pettee Gabriel, K., Zwald, M., Huberty, J., & Zhang, Y. (2009). Changes in psychosocial factors and physical activity frequency among third- to eighth-grade girls who participated in a developmentally focused youth sport program: A preliminary study. *The Journal of School Health*, 79(10), 474–484.

DeBate, R. D., & Thompson, S. H. (2005). Girls on the run: Improvements in self-esteem, body size satisfaction, and eating attitudes/behaviors. *Eating and Weight Disorders*, 10(1), 25–32.

Deci, E. L., & Ryan, R. M. (2000). The "what" and "why" of goal pursuits: Human needs and the self-determination of behavior. *Psychological Inquiry*, 11(4), 227–268.

de Morree, H. M., Klein, C., & Marcora, S. M. (2012). Perception of effort reflects central motor command during movement execution. *Psychophysiology*, 49(9), 1242–1253.

De Petrillo, L. A., Kaufman, K. A., Glass, C. R., & Arnkoff, D. B. (2009). Mindfulness for long-distance runners: An open trial using mindful sport performance enhancement (MPSE). *Journal of Clinical Sport Psychology*, 3(4), 357–376.

DeWolfe, C. E. J., Scott, D., & Seaman, K. A. (2021). Embrace the challenge: Acknowledging a challenge following negative self-talk improves performance. *Journal of Applied Sport Psychology*, 33(5), 527–540.

Dietrich, A., & McDaniel, W. F. (2004). Endocannabinoids and exercise. *British Journal of Sports Medicine*, 38(5), 536–541.

Donohue, B., Barnhart, R., Covassin, T., Carpin, K., & Korb, E. (2001). The development and initial evaluation of two promising mental preparatory methods in a sample of female cross-country runners. *Journal of Sport Behavior*, 24, 19–30.

Doose, M., Ziegenbein, M., Hoos, O., Reim, D., Stengert, W., Hoffer, N., Vogel, C., Ziert, Y., & Sieberer, M. (2015). Self-selected intensity exercise in the treatment of major depression: A pragmatic RCT. *International Journal of Psychiatry and Clinical Practice*, 19, 266–275.

Dring, K. J., Hatch, L. M., Williams, R. A., Morris, J. G., Sunderland, C., Nevill, M. E., & Cooper, S. B. (2022). Effect of 5-weeks participation in The Daily Mile on cognitive function, physical fitness, and body composition in children. *Scientific Reports*, 12(1), 14309.

Dunne, A., Haake, S., Quirk, H., & Bullas, A. (2021). Motivation to improve mental wellbeing via community physical activity initiatives and the associated impacts-a cross-sectional survey of UK parkrun participants. *International Journal of Environmental Research and Public Health*, 18(24), 13072.

Egorov, A. Y., & Szabo, A. (2013). The exercise paradox: An interactional model for a clearer conceptualization of exercise addiction. *Journal of Behavioral Addictions*, 2(4), 199–208.

Ekkekakis, P., Parfitt, G., & Petruzzello, S. J. (2011). The pleasure and displeasure people feel when they exercise at different intensities: Decennial update and progress towards a tripartite rationale for exercise intensity prescription. *Sports Medicine*, 41(8), 641–671.

Fabel, K., Fabel, K., Tam, B., Kaufer, D., Baiker, A., Simmons, N., Kuo, C. J., & Palmer, T. D. (2003). VEGF is necessary for exercise-induced adult hippocampal neurogenesis. *The European Journal of Neuroscience*, 18(10), 2803–2812.

Filby, W. C. D., Maynard, I. W., & Graydon, J. K. (1999). The effect of multiple-goal strategies on performance outcomes in training and competition. *Journal of Applied Sport Psychology*, 11, 230–246.

Filo, K., Funk, D. C., & O'Brien, D. (2011). Examining motivation for charity sport event participation: A comparison of recreation-based and charity-based motives. *Journal of Leisure Research*, 43(4), 491–518.

Fleming, J., Wellington, C., Parsons, J., & Dale, J. (2022). Collaboration between primary care and a voluntary, community sector organisation: Practical guidance from the parkrun practice initiative. *Health and Social Care in the Community*, 30(2), e514–e523.

Fokkema, T., Hartgens, F., Kluitenberg, B., Verhagen, E., Backx, F. J. G., van der Worp, H., Bierma-Zeinstra, S. M. A., Koes, B. W., & van Middelkoop, M. (2019). Reasons and predictors of discontinuation of running after a running program for novice runners. *Journal of Science and Medicine in Sport*, 22(1), 106–111.

Freimuth, M., Moniz, S., & Kim, S. R. (2011). Clarifying exercise addiction: Differential diagnosis, co-occurring disorders, and phases of addiction. *International Journal of Environmental Research and Public Health*, 8(10), 4069–4081.

Freund, W., Weber, F., Billich, C., Birklein, F., Breimhorst, M., & Schuetz, U. H. (2013). Ultra-marathon runners are different: Investigations into pain tolerance and personality traits of participants of the TransEurope FootRace 2009. *Pain Practice: The Official Journal of World Institute of Pain*, 13(7), 524–532.

Gattoni, C., O'Neill, B. V., Tarperi, C., Schena, F., & Marcora, S. M. (2021). The effect of mental fatigue on half-marathon performance: A pragmatic trial. *Sport Science and Health*, 17, 807–816.

Giles, G. E., Cantelon, J. A., Eddy, M. D., Brunyé, T. T., Urry, H. L., Taylor, H. A., Mahoney, C. R., & Kanarek, R. B. (2018). Cognitive reappraisal reduces perceived exertion during endurance exercise. *Motivation and Emotion*, 42, 482–496.

Gollwitzer, P. M. (1999). Implementation intentions: Strong effects of simple plans. *American Psychologist*, 54, 493–503.

Goodsell, T. L., Harris, B. D., & Bailey, B. W. (2013). Family status and motivations to run: A qualitative study of marathon runners. *Leisure Sciences: An Interdisciplinary Journal*, 35(4), 337–352.

Griffiths, M. D., Szabo, A., & Terry, A. (2005). The exercise addiction inventory: A quick and easy screening tool for health practitioners. *British Journal of Sports Medicine*, 39, e30.

Grunseit, A. C., Richards, J., Reece, L., Bauman, A., & Merom, D. (2020). Evidence on the reach and impact of the social physical activity phenomenon parkrun: A scoping review. *Preventive Medicine Reports*, 20, 101231.

Haake, S., Quick, H., & Bullas, A. (2022). Parkrun as a tool to support public health: Insights for clinicians. *British Journal of General Practice*. https://shura.shu.ac.uk/30407/

Hamer, M., Karageorghis, C. I., & Vlachopoulos, S. P. (2002). Motives for exercise participation as predictors of exercise dependence among endurance athletes. *The Journal of Sports Medicine and Physical Fitness*, 42, 233–238.

Hammer, C., & Podlog, L. (2016). Motivation and marathon running. In C. Zinner & B. Sperlich (Eds.), *Marathon running: Physiology, psychology, nutrition and training aspects* (pp. 107–124). Springer.

Hardy, C. J., & Rejeski, W. J. (1989). Not what, but how one feels: The measurement of affect during exercise. *Journal of Sport and Exercise Psychology*, 11, 304–317.

Hardy, C. J., Thomas, A. V., & Blanchfield, A. W. (2019). To me to you: How you say things matters for endurance performance. *Journal of Sports Science*, 37(18), 2122–2130.

Harte, J. L., & Eifert, G. H. (1995). The effects of running, environment, and attentional focus on athletes' catecholamine and cortisol levels and mood. *Psychophysiology*, 32, 49–54.

Hatzigeorgiadis, A., Bartura, K., Argiropoulos, C., Comoutos, N., Galanis, E., & Flouris, A. D. (2018). Beat the heat: Effects of a motivational self-talk intervention on endurance performance. *Journal of Applied Sport Psychology*, 30, 388–401.

Hawkins, R. M., Crust, L., Swann, C., & Jackman, P. C. (2020). The effects of goal types on psychological outcomes in active and insufficiently active adults in a walking task: Further evidence for open goals. *Psychology of Sport and Exercise*, 48, 101661.

Heijnen, S., Hommel, B., Kibele, A., & Colzato, L. S. (2016). Neuromodulation of aerobic exercise-a review. *Frontiers in Psychology*, 6, 1890.

Herring, M. P., Lindheimer, J. B., & O'Connor, P. J. (2014). The effects of exercise training on anxiety. *American Journal of Lifestyle Medicine*, 8(6), 388–403.

Hill, A., Schücker, L., Hagemann, N., & Strauss, B. (2017). Further evidence for an external focus of attention in running: Looking at specific focus instructions and individual differences. *Journal of Sport and Exercise Psychology*, 39(5), 352–365.

Hindley, D. (2020). "More than just a run in the park": An exploration of parkrun as a shared leisure space. *Leisure Sciences*, 42(1), 85–105.

Hut, M., Minkler, T. O., Glass, C. R., Weppner, C. H., Thomas, H. M., & Flannery, C. B. (2021). A randomized controlled study of mindful sport performance enhancement and psychological skills training with collegiate track and field athletes. *Journal of Applied Sport Psychology*, Advance online publication.

Hutchinson, J. C., Jones, L., Vitti, S. N., Moore, A., Dalton, P. C., & O'Neil, B. J. (2018). The influence of self-selected music on affect-regulated exercise intensity and remembered pleasure during treadmill running. *Sport, Exercise, and Performance Psychology*, 7(1), 80–92.

Hutchinson, J. C., & Karageorghis, C. I. (2013). Moderating influence of dominant attentional style and exercise intensity on responses to asynchronous music. *Journal of Sport and Exercise Psychology*, 35(6), 625–643.

Inoue, Y., Funk, D., & Jordan, J. S. (2013). The role of running involvement in creating self-sufficiency for homeless individuals through a community-based running programme. *Journal of Sport Management*, 27, 439–452.

Jackman, P. C., Brick, N. E., Whitehead, A. E., & Swann, C. (in press). Goal setting and goal striving in excellent running performances: A qualitative exploration. *Psychology of Sport and Exercise*.

Jackman, P. C., Hawkins, R. M., Whitehead, A. E., & Brick, N. E. (2021). Integrating models of self-regulation and optimal experiences: A qualitative study into flow and clutch states in recreational distance running. *Psychology of Sport and Exercise*, 57, 102051.

Joyner, M. J., & Coyle, E. F. (2008). Endurance exercise performance: The physiology of champions. *Journal of Physiology*, 586, 35–44.

Joyner, M. J., Hunter, S. K., Lucia, A., & Jones, A. M. (2020). Physiology and fast marathons. *Journal of Applied Physiology*, 128(4), 1065–1068.

Kalak, N., Gerber, M., Kirov, R., Mikoteit, T., Yordanova, J., Pühse, U., Holsboer-Trachsler, E., & Brand, S. (2012). Daily morning running for 3 weeks improved sleep and psychological functioning in healthy adolescents compared with controls. *The Journal of Adolescent Health: Official Publication of the Society for Adolescent Medicine, 51*(6), 615–622.

Karageorghis, C. I., & Priest, D. L. (2012a). Music in the exercise domain: A review and synthesis (Part I). *International Review of Sport and Exercise Psychology, 5*(1), 44–66.

Karageorghis, C. I., & Priest, D. L. (2012b). Music in the exercise domain: A review and synthesis (Part II). *International Review of Sport and Exercise Psychology, 5*(1), 67–84.

Kaufman, K. A., Glass, C. R., & Arnkoff, D. B. (2009). Evaluation of mindful sport performance enhancement (MPSE): A new approach to promote flow in athletes. *Journal of Clinical Sport Psychology, 3*(4), 334–356.

Keating, L. E., Becker, S., McCabe, K., Whattam, J., Garrick, L., Sassi, R. B., Frey, B. N., & McKinnon, M. C. (2018). Effects of a 12-week running programme in youth and adults with complex mood disorders. *BMJ Open Sport and Exercise Medicine, 4*(1), e000314.

Kerr, J. H., Fujiyama, H., Sugano, A., Okamura, T., Chang, M., & Onouha, F. (2006). Psychological responses to exercising in laboratory and natural environments. *Psychology of Sport and Exercise, 7*(4), 345–359.

Kramer, A. F., & Colcombe, S. (2018). Fitness effects on the cognitive function of older adults: A meta-analytic study revisited. *Perspectives on Psychological Science, 13*(2), 213–221.

Krouse, R. Z., Ransdell, L. B., Lucas, S. M., & Pritchard, M. E. (2011). Motivation, goal orientation, coaching, and training habits of women ultrarunners. *Journal of Strength and Conditioning Research, 25*(10), 2835–2842.

Kruisdijk, F. R., Hendriksen, I. J., Tak, E. C., Beekman, A. T., & Hopman-Rock, M. (2012). Effect of running therapy on depression (EFFORT-D). Design of a randomised controlled trial in adult patients [ISRCTN 1894]. *BMC Public Health, 12*, 50.

Kyllo, L. B., & Landers, D. M. (1995). Goal setting in sport and exercise: A research synthesis to resolve the controversy. *Journal of Sport and Exercise Psychology, 17*(2), 117–137.

LaCaille, R. A., Masters, K. S., & Heath, E. M. (2004). Effects of cognitive strategy and exercise setting on running performance, perceived exertion, affect, and satisfaction. *Psychology of Sport and Exercise, 5*, 461–476.

Lane, A. M., Devonport, T. J., Friesen, A. P., Beedie, C. J., Fullerton, C. L., & Stanley, D. M. (2016a). How should I regulate my emotions if I want to run faster? *European Journal of Sports Science, 16*(4), 465–472.

Lane, A. M., Devonport, T. J., Stanley, D. M., & Beedie, C. J. (2016b). The effects of brief online self-help intervention strategies on emotions and satisfaction with running performance. *Sensoria: A Journal of Mind, Brain and Culture, 12*(2), 30–39.

Lane, A. M., Murphy, N. M., & Bauman, A. (2008). *The impact of participation in the Flora women's mini-marathon on physical activity behaviour in women. Research report 1.* Centre for Health Behaviour Research, Department of Health Sport and Exercise Sciences, Waterford Institute of Technology and Irish Sports Council.

Lane, A. M., Terry, P. C., & Karageorghis, C. I. (1995). Path analysis examining relationships among antecedents of anxiety, multidimensional state anxiety, and triathlon performance. *Perceptual and Motor Skills, 81*(Suppl 3), 1255–1266.

Larumbe-Zabala, E., Esteve-Lanao, J., Cardona, C. A., Alcocer, A., & Quartiroli, A. (2020). Longitudinal analysis of marathon runners' psychological state and its relationship with running speed at ventilatory thresholds. *Frontiers in Psychology, 11,* 545.

Lasnier, J., & Durand-Bush, N. (2022). How elite endurance athletes experience and manage exercise-induced pain: Implications for mental performance consultants. *Journal of Applied Sport Psychology,* Advance Online Publication.

Latinjak, A. T., Hatzigeorgiadis, A., Comoutos, N., & Hardy, J. (2019). Speaking clearly . . . 10 years on: The case for an integrative perspective of self-talk in sport. *Sport and Exercise Performance Psychology, 8,* 353–367.

León-Guereño, P., Tapia-Serrano, M. A., Castañeda-Babarro, A., & Malchrowicz-Mos'ko, E. (2020). Do sex, age, and marital status influence the motivations of amateur marathon runners? The Poznan marathon case study. *Frontiers in Psychology, 11,* 2151.

Lerner, R. M., Lerner, J. V., Almerigi, J. B., Theokas, C., Phelps, E., Gestsdottir, S., Naudeau, S., Jelicic, H., Alberts, A., Ma, L., Smith, L. M., Bobek, D. L., Richman-Raphael, D., Simpson, I., Christiansen, E. D., & von Eye, A. (2005). Positive youth development, participation in community youth development programs, and community contributions of fifth-grade adolescents: Findings from the first wave of the 4-H study of positive youth development. *The Journal of Early Adolescence, 25*(1), 17–71.

Lieberman, D. E. (2011). *The evolution of the human head.* Harvard University Press.

Lieberman, D. E., Bramble, D. M., Raichlen, D. A., & Shea, J. J. (2006). Brains, brawn, and the evolution of human endurance running capabilities. In F. E. Grine, J. G. Fleagle, & R. L. Leakey (Eds.), *The first humans: Origin and early evolution of the genus homo* (pp. 77–92). Springer.

Lind, E., Welch, A. S., & Ekkekakis, P. (2009). Do 'mind over muscle' strategies work? *Sports Medicine, 39,* 743–764.

Locke, E. A., & Latham, G. P. (1985). The application of goal setting to sports. *Journal of Sport Psychology, 7*(3), 205–222.

Maceri, R. M., Cherup, N. P., Buckworth, J., & Hanson, N. J. (2021). Exercise addiction in long distance runners. *International Journal of Mental Health Addiction, 19,* 62–71.

MacMahon, C., Schücker, L., Hagemann, N., & Strauss, B. (2014). Cognitive fatigue effects on physical performance during running. *Journal of Sport and Exercise Psychology, 36*(4), 375–381.

Maehr, M. L., & Zusho, A. (2009). Achievement goal theory: The past, present, and future. In K. R. Wenzel & A. Wigfield (Eds.), *Handbook of motivation at school* (pp. 77–104). Routledge.

Malchrowicz-Mośko, E., León-Guereño, P., Tapia-Serrano, M. A., Sánchez-Miguel, P. A., & Waśkiewicz, Z. (2020). What encourages physically inactive people to start running? an analysis of motivations to participate in parkrun and city trail in Poland. *Frontiers in Public Health. 8,* 581017.

Marcora, S. M. (2010). Counterpoint: Afferent feedback from fatigued locomotor muscles is not an important determinant of endurance exercise performance. *Journal of Applied Physiology, 108,* 454–456.

Marcora, S. M. (2019). Psychobiology of fatigue during endurance performance. In C. Meijen (Ed.), *Endurance performance in sport: Psychological theory and interventions* (pp. 15–34). Routledge.

Marcora, S. M., & Staiano, W. (2010). The limit to exercise tolerance in humans: Mind over muscle? *European Journal of Applied Physiology, 109*(4), 763–770.

Marcora, S. M., Staiano, W., & Manning, V. (2009). Mental fatigue impairs physical performance in humans. *Journal of Applied Physiology, 106*(3), 857–864.

Markowitz, S. M., & Arent, S. M. (2010). The exercise and affect relationship: Evidence for the dual-mode model and a modified opponent process theory. *Journal of Sport and Exercise Psychology, 32*(5), 711–730.

Martin, J. J., Waldron, J. J., McCabe, A., & Choi, Y. S. (2009). The impact of "girls on the run" on self-concept and fat attitudes. *Journal of Clinical Sport Psychology, 3*(2), 127–138.

Martin, K., Meeusen, R., Thompson, K. G., Keegan, R., & Rattay, B. (2018). Mental fatigue impairs endurance performance: A physiological explanation. *Sports Medicine*, 48, 2041–2051.

Martin, K., Staiano, W., Menaspà, P., Hennessey, T., Marcora, S., Keegan, R., Thompson, K. G., Martin, D., Halson, S., & Rattray, B. (2016). Superior inhibitory control and resistance to mental fatigue in professional road cyclists. *PLoS One*, 11(7), e0159907.

Masters, K. S., & Ogles, B. M. (1995). An investigation of the different motivations of marathon runners with varying degrees of experience. *Journal of Sport Behaviour*, 18(1), 69–79.

Masters, K. S., & Ogles, B. M. (1998). Associative and dissociative cognitive strategies in exercise and running: 20 years later what do we know? *The Sport Psychologist*, 12, 253–270.

Masters, K. S., Ogles, B. M., & Jolton, J. A. (1993). The development of an instrument to measure motivation for marathon running: The motivations of marathoners scales (MOMS). *Research Quarterly for Exercise and Sport*, 64(2), 134–143.

Mauger, A. R. (2019). Exercise-induced pain: A psychophysiological perspective. In C. Meijen (Ed.), *Endurance performance in sport: Psychological theory and interventions* (pp. 35–46). Routledge.

McCallie, M. S., Blum, C. M., & Hood, C. J. (2006). Progressive muscle relaxation. *Journal of Human Behavior in the Social Environment*, 13(3), 51–66.

McCormick, A., Meijen, C., & Marcora, S. (2018). Effects of a motivational self-talk intervention for endurance athletes completing an ultramarathon. *The Sport Psychologist*, 32, 42–50.

McDowell, C. P., Campbell, M. J., & Herring, M. P. (2016). Sex-related differences in mood responses to acute aerobic exercise. *Medicine and Science in Sports and Exercise*, 48(9), 1798–1802.

McNamara, J., & McCabe, M. P. (2013). Development and validation of the exercise dependence and elite athletes scale. *Performance Enhancement and Health*, 2(1), 30–36.

Meijen, C., Day, C., & Hays, K. F. (2017). Running a psyching team: Providing mental support at long-distance running events. *Journal of Sport Psychology in Action*, 8, 12–22.

Meijen, C., McCormick, A., Anstiss, P. A., & Marcora, S. M. (2021). "Short and sweet": A randomized controlled initial investigation of brief online psychological interventions with endurance athletes. *The Sport Psychologist*, 36, 20–28.

Miller, A., & Donohue, B. (2003). The development and controlled evaluation of athletic mental preparation strategies in high school distance runners. *Journal of Applied Sport Psychology*, 15, 321–334.

Mónok, K., Berczik, K., Urbán, R., Szabó, A., Griffiths, M. D., Farkas, J., Magi, A., Eisinger, A., Kurimay, T., Kökönyei, G., Kun, B., Paksi, B., & Demetrovics, Z. (2012). Psychometric properties and concurrent validity of two exercise addiction measures: A population wide study in Hungary. *Psychology of Sport and Exercise*, 13, 739–746.

Morgan, W. P., & Pollock, M. L. (1977). Psychologic characterization of the elite distance runner. *Annals of the New York Academy of Sciences*, 301, 382–403.

Morris, P., & Scott, H. (2019). Not just a run in the park: A qualitative exploration of parkrun and mental health. *Advances in Mental Health*, 17(2), 110–123.

Moses, J., Steptoe, A., Mathews, A., & Edwards, S. (1989). The effects of exercise training on mental well-being in the normal population: A controlled trial. *Journal of Psychometric Research*, 33(1), 47–61.

Nettleton, S., & Hardey, M. (2006). Running away with health: The urban marathon and the construction of 'charitable bodies'. *Health (London)*, 10(4), 441–460.

Nezlek, J. B., Cypryańska, M., Cypryański, P., Chlebosz, K., Jenczylik, K., Sztachańska, J., & Zalewska, A. M. (2018). Within-person relationships between recreational running and psychological well-being. *Journal of Sport and Exercise Psychology*, 40(3), 146–152.

Nikol, L., Kuan, G., Ong, M., Chang, Y.-K., & Terry, P. C. (2018). The heat is on: Effects of synchronous music on psychophysiological parameters and running performance in hot and humid conditions. *Frontiers in Psychology*, 9, 1114.

Noakes, T., St Clair Gibson, A., & Lambert, E. V. (2005). From catastrophe to complexity: A novel model of integrative central neural regulation of effort and fatigue during exercise in humans: Summary and conclusions. *British Journal of Sports Medicine*, 39(2), 120–124.

O'Connor, P. J., & Cook, D. B. (1999). Exercise and pain: The neurobiology, measurement, and laboratory study of pain in relation to exercise in humans. *Exercise and Sport Sciences Reviews*, 27, 119–166.

Oettingen, G. (2012). Future thought and behaviour change. *European Review of Social Psychology*, 23, 1–63.

Ogles, B. M., & Masters, K. S. (2003). A typology of marathon runners based on cluster analysis of motivations. *Journal of Sport Behavior*, 26(1), 69–85.

O'Leary, T. J., Collett, J., Howells, K., & Morris, M. G. (2017). High but not moderate-intensity endurance training increases pain tolerance: A randomised trial. *European Journal of Applied Physiology*, 117(11), 2201–2210.

Oswald, F., Campbell, J., Williamson, C., Richards, J., & Kelly, P. (2020). A scoping review of the relationship between running and mental health. *International Journal of Environmental Research and Public Health*, 17(21), 8059.

Pageaux, B. (2016). Perception of effort in exercise science: Definition, measurement and perspectives. *European Journal of Sport Science*, 16(8), 885–894.

Pageaux, B., Lepers, R., Dietz, K. C., & Marcora, S. M. (2014). Response inhibition impairs subsequent self-paced endurance performance. *European Journal of Applied Physiology*, 114(5), 1095–1105.

Patrick, T. D., & Hrycaiko, D. W. (1998). Effects of a mental training package on an endurance performance. *The Sport Psychologist*, 12, 283–299.

Pedisic, Z., Shrestha, N., Kovalchik, S., Stamatakis, E., Liangruenrom, N., Grgic, J., Titze, S., Biddle, S. J., Bauman, A. E., & Oja, P. (2020). Is running associated with a lower risk of all-cause, cardiovascular and cancer mortality, and is the more the better? A systematic review and meta-analysis. *British Journal of Sports Medicine*, 54, 898–905.

Peterson, B., Withers, B., Hawke, F., Spink, M., Callister, R., & Chuter, V. (2022). Outcomes of participation in parkrun, and factors influencing why and how often individuals participate: A systematic review of quantitative studies. *Journal of Sports Sciences*, 40(13), 1486–1499.

Pettee Gabriel, K. K., DiGioacchino DeBate, R., High, R. R., & Racine, E. F. (2011). Girls on the run: A quasi-experimental evaluation of a developmentally focused youth sport program. *Journal of Physical Activity and Health*, 8(Suppl 2), S285–S294.

Poczta, J., Malchrowicz-Mo´sko, E., & Braga de Melo Fadigas, A. (2018). Age-related motives in mass running events participation. *Olimpianos— Journal of Olympic Studies*, 2(1), 257–273.

Pollak, K. A., Swenson, J. D., Vanhaitsma, T. A., Hughen, R. W., Jo, D., White, A. T., Light, K. C., Schweinhardt, P., Amann, M., & Light, A. R. (2014). Exogenously applied muscle metabolites synergistically evoke sensations of muscle fatigue and pain in human subjects. *Experimental Physiology*, 99(2), 368–380.

Raichlen, D. A., & Alexander, G. E. (2017). Adaptive capacity: An evolutionary neuroscience model linking exercise, cognition, and brain health. *Trends in Neurosciences*, 40(7), 408–421.

Raichlen, D. A., Foster, A. D., Gerdeman, G. L., Seillier, A., & Giuffrida, A. (2012). Wired to run: Exercise-induced endocannabinoid signaling in humans and cursorial mammals with implications for the 'runner's high'. *The Journal of Experimental Biology*, 215(Pt 8), 1331–1336.

Raichlen, D. A., Foster, A. D., Seillier, A., Giuffrida, A., & Gerdeman, G. L. (2013). Exercise-induced endocannabinoid signaling is modulated by intensity. *European Journal of Applied Physiology*, 113(4), 869–875.

Ram, B., Chalkley, A., van Sluijs, E., Phillips, R., Venkatraman, T., Hargreaves, D. S., Viner, R. M., & Saxena, S. (2021). Impact of The Daily Mile on children's physical and mental health, and educational attainment in primary schools: Improve cohort study protocol. *BMJ Open*, 11(5), e045879.

Rebar, A. L., Faulkner, G., & Stanton, R. (2015). An exploratory study examining the core affect hypothesis of the anti-depressive and anxiolytic effects of physical activity. *Mental Health and Physical Activity*, 9, 55–58.

Reed, J., & Buck, S. (2009). The effect of regular aerobic exercise on positive-activated affect: A meta-analysis. *Psychology of Sport and Exercise*, 10(6), 581–594.

Reed, J., & Ones, D. S. (2006). The effect of acute aerobic exercise on positive activated affect: A meta-analysis. *Psychology of Sport and Exercise*, 7, 477–514.

Riddell, H., Lamont, W., Lombard, M., Paduano, S., Maltagliati, S., Gucciardi, D. F., & Ntoumanis, N. (2023). Autonomous motivation promotes goal attainment through the conscious investment of effort, but mental contrasting with implementation intentions makes goal striving easier. *The Journal of Social Psychology*, 1–14. Advance online publication.

Rizzo, N. (2021). 120+ Running statistics 2021/2022 [Research review]. https://runrepeat.com/running-statistics

Roebuck, G. S., Fitzgerald, P. B., Urquhart, D. M., Ng, S. N., Cicuttini, F. M., & Fitzgibbon, B. M. (2018). The psychology of ultra-marathon runners: A systematic review. *Psychology of Sport and Exercise*, 37, 43–58.

Rogerson, M., Brown, D. K., Sandercock, G., Wooller, J. J., & Barton, J. (2016). A comparison of four typical green exercise environments and prediction of psychological health outcomes. *Perspectives in Public Health*, 136(3), 171–180.

Rolian, C., Lieberman, D. E., Hamill, J., Scott, J. W., & Werbel, W. (2009). Walking, running and the evolution of short toes in humans. *The Journal of Experimental Biology*, 212(5), 713–721.

Rozmiarek, M., Malchrowicz-Mo´sko, E., León-Guereño, P., Tapia-Serrano, M. Á., & Kwiatkowski, G. (2021). Motivational differences between 5k runners, marathoners and ultramarathoners in Poland. *Sustainability*, 13, 6980.

Sachs, M. L., & Pargman, D. (1984). Running addiction. In M. L. Sachs & G. W. Buffone (Eds.), *Running as therapy: An integrated approach* (pp. 231–252). University of Nebraska Press.

Samson, A. (2014). Sources of self-efficacy during marathon training: A qualitative, longitudinal investigation. *The Sport Psychologist*, 28, 164–175.

Scheerder, J., Breedveld, K., & Borgers, J. (2015). Who is doing a run with the running boom? The growth and governance of one of Europe's most popular sport activities. In J. Scheerder, K. Breedveld, & J. Borgers (Eds.), *Running across Europe: The rise and size of one of the largest sports markets* (pp. 1–27). Palgrave Macmillan.

Schomer, H. H. (1986). Mental strategies and the perception of effort of marathon runners. *International Journal of Sport Psychology*, 17, 41–59.

Schomer, H. H. (1987). Mental strategy training programme for marathon runners. *International Journal of Sport Psychology*, 18, 133–151.

Schuch, F. B., Vancampfort, D., Richards, J., Rosenbaum, S., Ward, P. B., & Stubbs, B. (2016). Exercise as a treatment for depression: A meta-analysis adjusting for publication bias. *Journal of Psychiatric Research*, 77, 42–51.

Schücker, L., Knopf, C., Strauss, B., & Hagemann, N. (2014). An internal focus of attention is not always as bad as its reputation: How specific aspects of internally focused attention do not hinder running efficiency. *Journal of Sport and Exercise Psychology*, 36, 223–243.

Schüler, J., & Langens, T. A. (2007). Psychological crisis in a marathon and the buffering effects of self-verbalizations. *Journal of Applied Social Psychology*, 37, 2319–2344.

Shannon, S., Shevlin, M., Brick, N., & Breslin, G. (2023). Frequency, intensity and duration of muscle strengthening activity and associations with mental health. *Journal of Affective Disorders*, 325, 41–47.

Sifers, S. K., & Shea, D. N. (2013). Evaluation of girls on the run/girls on track to enhance self-esteem and well-being. *Journal of Clinical Sport Psychology*, 7, 77–85.

Simpson, S. D., & Karageorghis, C. I. (2006). The effects of synchronous music on 400-m sprint performance. *Journal of Sports Sciences*, 24, 1095–1102.

Smith, A. L., Gill, D. L., Crews, D. J., Hopewell, R., & Morgan, D. W. (1995). Attentional strategy use by experienced distance runners: Physiological and psychological effects. *Research Quarterly in Exercise and Sport*, 66, 142–150.

Smith, D., Wright, C., & Winrow, D. (2010). Exercise dependence and social physique anxiety in competitive and non-competitive runners. *International Journal of Sport and Exercise Psychology*, 8(1), 61–69.

Sparling, P. B., Giuffrida, A., Piomelli, D., Rosskopf, L., & Dietrich, A. (2003). Exercise activates the endocannabinoid system. *Neuroreport*, 14(17), 2209–2211.

Spoor, F., Wood, B., & Zonneveld, F. (1994). Implications of early hominid labyrinthine morphology for evolution of human bipedal locomotion. *Nature*, 369, 645–648.

Stanley, D. M., & Cumming, J. (2010a). Are we having fun yet? Testing the effects of imagery use on the affective and enjoyment responses to acute moderate exercise. *Psychology of Sport and Exercise*, 11, 582–590.

Stanley, D. M., & Cumming, J. (2010b). Not just how one feels, but what one images? The effects of imagery use on affective responses to moderate exercise. *International Journal of Sport and Exercise Psychology*, 8(4), 343–359.

Stanley, D. M., Lane, A. M., Beedie, C. J., Friesen, A. P., & Devonport, T. J. (2012). Emotion regulation strategies used in the hour before running. *International Journal of Sport and Exercise Psychology*, 10, 159–171.

Stevinson, C. D., & Biddle, S. J. H. (1998). Cognitive orientations in marathon running and 'hitting the wall'. *British Journal of Sports Medicine*, 32, 229–235.

Stevinson, C., & Hickson, M. (2019). Changes in physical activity, weight and wellbeing outcomes among attendees of a weekly mass participation event: A prospective 12-month study. *Journal of Public Health (Oxford, England)*, 41(4), 807–814.

Svebak, S., & Murgatoyd, S. (1985). Metamotivational dominance: A multitimethod validation of reversal theory constructs. *Journal of Personality and Social Psychology*, 48, 107–116.

Swann, C., Hooper, A., Schweickle, M. J., Peoples, G., Mullan, J., Hutto, D., Allen, M. S., & Vella, S. A. (2020). Comparing the effects of goal types in a walking session with healthy adults: Preliminary evidence for open goals in physical activity. *Psychology of Sport and Exercise*, 47, 101475.

Szabo, A. (1995). The impact of exercise deprivation on well-being of habitual exercisers. *The Australian Journal of Science and Medicine in Sport*, 27, 68–75.

Szabo, A. (2003). The acute effects of humor and exercise on mood and anxiety. *Journal of Leisure Research, 35*(2), 152–162.

Szabo, A., & Egorov, A. Y. (2016). Exercise addiction. In A. M. Lane (Ed.), *Sport and exercise psychology* (2nd ed., pp. 178–210). Routledge.

Szmedra, L., & Bacharach, D. W. (1998). Effect of music on perceived exertion, plasma lactate, norepinephrine and cardiovascular hemodynamics during treadmill running. *International Journal of Sports Medicine, 19,* 32–37.

Teixeira, P. J., Carraça, E. V., Markland, D., Silva, M. N., & Ryan, R. M. (2012). Exercise, physical activity, and self-determination theory: A systematic review. *The International Journal of Behavioral Nutrition and Physical Activity, 9,* 78.

Tempest, G. D., & Parfitt, G. (2013). Imagery use and affective responses during exercise: An examination of cerebral hemodynamics using near-infrared spectroscopy. *Journal of Sport and Exercise Psychology, 35*(5), 503–513.

Tenenbaum, G. (2001). A social-cognitive perspective of perceived exertion and exertion tolerance. In R. N. Singer, H. A. Hausenblas, & C. Janelle (Eds.), *Handbook of sport psychology* (pp. 810–822). Wiley.

Tenenbaum, G., Lidor, R., Lavyan, N., Morrow, K., Tonnel, S., Gershgoren, A., Meis, J., & Johnson, M. (2004). The effect of music type on running perseverance and coping with effort sensations. *Psychology of Sport and Exercise, 5*(2), 89–109.

Tenenbaum, G., Spence, R., & Christensen, S. (1999). The effect of goal difficulty and goal orientation on running performance in young female athletes. *Austalian Journal of Psychology, 51,* 6–11.

Terry, A., Szabo, A., & Griffiths, M. D. (2004). The exercise addiction inventory: A new brief screening tool. *Addiction Research and Theory, 12,* 489–499.

Terry, P. C., & Karageorghis, C. I. (2006). Psychophysical effects of music in sport and exercise: An update on theory, research and application. In M. Katsikitis (Ed.), *Proceedings of the 2006 joint conference of the APS and the NZPS* (pp. 415–419). Australian Psychological Society.

Terry, P. C., Karageorghis, C. I., Curran, M. L., Martin, O. V., & Parsons-Smith, R. L. (2020). Effects of music in exercise and sport: A meta-analytic review. *Psychological Bulletin, 146*(2), 91–117.

Terry, P. C., Karageorghis, C. I., Saha, A. M., & D'Auria, S. (2012). Effects of synchronous music on treadmill running among elite triathletes. *Journal of Science and Medicine in Sport, 15*(1), 52–57.

Terry, P. C., Lane, A. M., & Fogarty, G. J. (2003). Construct validity of the profile of mood state—adolescents for use with adults. *Psychology of Sport and Exercise, 4*(2), 125–139.

Tesarz, J., Schuster, A. K., Hartmann, M., Gerhardt, A., & Eich, W. (2012). Pain perception in athletes compared to normally active controls: A systematic review with meta-analysis. *Pain, 153*(6), 1253–1262.

Thelwell, R. C., & Greenlees, I. A. (2001). The effects of a mental skills training package on gymnasium triathlon performance. *The Sport Psychologist, 5,* 127–141.

Thelwell, R. C., & Greenlees, I. A. (2003). Developing competitive endurance performance using mental skills training. *The Sport Psychologist, 17,* 318–337.

Thompson, R. W., Kaufman, K. A., de Petrillo, L. A., Glass, C. R., & Arnkoff, D. B. (2011). One year follow-up of mindful sport performance enhancement (MPSE) with archers, golfers, and runners. *Journal of Clinical Sport Psychology, 5,* 99–116.

Thornton, E. W., & Scott, S. E. (1995). Motivation in the committed runner: Correlations between self-report scales and behavior. *Health Promotion International, 10*(3), 177–184.

Tomporowski, P. D., McCullick, B., Pendleton, D. M., & Pesce, C. (2015). Exercise and children's cognition: The role of exercise characteristics and a place for metacognition. *Journal of Sport and Health Science, 4*(1), 47–55.

Van Cutsem, J., Marcora, S., De Pauw, K., Bailey, S., Meeusen, R., & Roelands, B. (2017). The effects of mental fatigue on physical performance: A systematic review. *Sports Medicine, 47*(8), 1569–1588.

van Dyck, D., Cardon, G., de Bourdeaudhuij, I., de Ridder, L., & Willem, A. (2017). Who participates in running events? Socio-demographic characteristics, psychosocial factors and barriers as correlates of non-participation—A pilot study in Belgium. *International Journal of Environmental Research and Public Health, 14*(11), 1315.

Venhorst, A., Micklewright, D. P., & Noakes, T. D. (2018a). Towards a three-dimensional framework of centrally regulated and goal-directed exercise behaviour: A narrative review. *British Journal of Sports Medicine, 52*(15), 957–966.

Venhorst., A., Micklewright, D. P., & Noakes, T. D. (2018b). The psychophysiological determinants of pacing behaviour and performance during prolonged endurance exercise: A performance level and competition outcome comparison. *Sports Medicine, 48*(10), 2387–2400.

Venhorst., A., Micklewright, D. P., & Noakes, T. D. (2018c). The psychophysiological regulation of pacing behaviour and performance fatigability during long-distance running with locomotor muscle fatigue and exercise-induced muscle damage in highly trained runners. *Sports Medicine—Open*, 4(1), 29.

Von Haaren, B., Haertel, S., Stumpp, J., Hey, S., & Ebner-Priemer, U. (2015). Reduced emotional stress reactivity to a real-life academic examination stressor in students participating in a 20-week aerobic exercise training: A randomised controlled trial using Ambulatory assessment. *Psychology of Sport and Exercise*, 20, 67075.

Waddington, E. E., & Heisz, J. J. (2023). Orienteering experts report more proficient spatial processing and memory across adulthood. *PLoS One*, 18(1), e0280435.

Wang, Y., Tian, J., & Yang, Q. (2021). On mindfulness training for promoting mental toughness in female college students in endurance exercise. *Evidence-Based Complementary and Alternative Medicine*, 5596111.

Warner, R., & Griffiths, M. D. (2006). A qualitative thematic analysis of exercise addiction: An exploratory study. *International Journal of Mental Health and Addiction*, 4, 13–26.

Weinstein, A. A., Deuster, P. A., Francis, J. L., Beadling, C., & Kop, W. J. (2010). The role of depression in short-term mood and fatigue responses to acute exercise. *International Journal of Behavioural Medicine*, 17, 51–57.

Weiss, M. R., Kipp, L. E., Phillips Reichter, A., & Bolter, N. D. (2020). Evaluating girls on the run in promoting positive youth development: Group comparisons on life skills transfer and social processes. *Pediatric Exercise Science*, 32, 172–182.

Weiss, M. R., Kipp, L. E., Phillips Reichter, A., Espinoza, S. M., & Bolter, N. D. (2019). Girls on the run: Impact of a physical activity youth development program on psychosocial and behavioral outcomes. *Pediatric Exercise Science*, 31(3), 330–340.

Williams, T., Krahenbuhl, G., & Morgan, D. (1991). Mood state and running economy in moderately trained male runners. *Medicine and Science in Sports and Exercise*, 23(6), 727–731.

Williamson, O., Swann, C., Bennett, K. J. M., Bird, M. D., Goddard, S. G., Schweickle, M. J., & Jackman, P. C. (2022). The performance and psychological effects of goal setting in sport: A systematic review and meta-analysis. *International Review of Sport and Exercise Psychology*. https://www.tandfonline.com/doi/full/10.1080/1750984X.2022.2116723

Wiltshire, G. R., Fullagar, S., & Stevinson, C. (2018). Exploring parkrun as a social context for collective health practices: Running with and against the moral imperatives of health responsibilisation. *Sociology of Health & Illness*, 40(1), 3–17.

Wulf, G., McNevin, N. H., & Shea, C. H. (2001). The automaticity of complex motor skill learning as a function of attentional focus. *Quarterly Journal of Experimental Psychology*, 54, 1143–1154.

Youngman, J., & Simpson, D. (2014). Risk of exercise addiction: A comparison of triathletes training for sprint-, Olympic-, half-ironman-, and Ironman-distance triathlons. *Journal of Clinical Sport Psychology*, 8, 19–37.

Zach, S., Xia, Y., Zeev, A., Arnon, M., Choresh, N., & Tenenbaum, G. (2017). Motivation dimensions for running a marathon: A new model emerging from the Motivation of Marathon Scale (MOMS). *Journal of Sport and Health Science*, 6(3), 302–310.

Printed in the United States
by Baker & Taylor Publisher Services